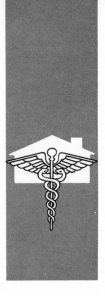

THE NEW ILLUSTRATED

MEDICAL ENCYCLOPEDIA

FOR HOME USE

VOLUME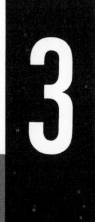

Compiled and Edited

ILLUSTRATED BY SYLVIA AND LESTER V. BERGMAN

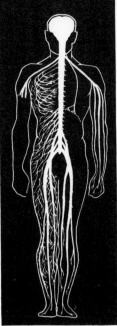

The *NEW* Illustrated
MEDICAL
ENCYCLOPEDIA
FOR HOME USE

A PRACTICAL GUIDE TO GOOD HEALTH

ROBERT E. ROTHENBERG, M.D., F.A.C.S.

ABRADALE PRESS *Publishers / New York*

NOTE TO THE READER

The reader is advised that for disorders requiring individual examination and treatment, a doctor must be consulted, for no prescription or course of treatment is intended to be recommended in these volumes.

NEWLY REVISED EDITION

Eighth Printing, September, 1963

DESIGNED BY HOWARD MORRIS
PRINTED IN THE UNITED STATES OF AMERICA

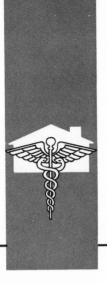

Table of Contents

This Table of Contents lists all topics in this particular volume only. For a complete Table of Contents listing all topics in the entire four volumes of this *New Illustrated Medical Encyclopedia*, see Volume One. A special section of Definitions of Common Medical Terms will be found at the end of Volume Four.

vii

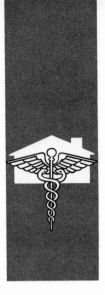

THE NEW ILLUSTRATED

MEDICAL ENCYCLOPEDIA

FOR HOME USE

CHAPTER **33**

The Kidneys
and Ureters

What is the location and structure of the kidneys?

The kidneys are two bean-shaped, reddish-brown organs covered by a glistening, thin capsule. Each kidney measures approximately four inches in length, two inches in width, and approximately one and one-half inches in thickness.

The kidneys lie on either side of the posterior portion of the abdomen, high up in the loin, behind the abdominal cavity and beneath the diaphragm.

How do the kidneys function?

The kidneys are composed of hundreds of thousands of tiny units known as nephrons, which empty into microscopic ducts known as tubules. Each nephron is a small independent chemical plant which forms urine as the plasma of the blood passes through. The nephrons empty the urine they produce into collecting tubules and then on into the pelvis of the kidney; thence, via a tubular structure called the ureter, into the urinary bladder.

What are the main duties of the kidneys?

Approximately one-fourth of the blood output of the heart is conveyed to the kidneys. The nephrons extract waste and toxic chemicals, excess minerals, and water from the blood which passes through them. It is also the function of the kidney *not to extract* certain needed chemicals and substances from the blood.

712

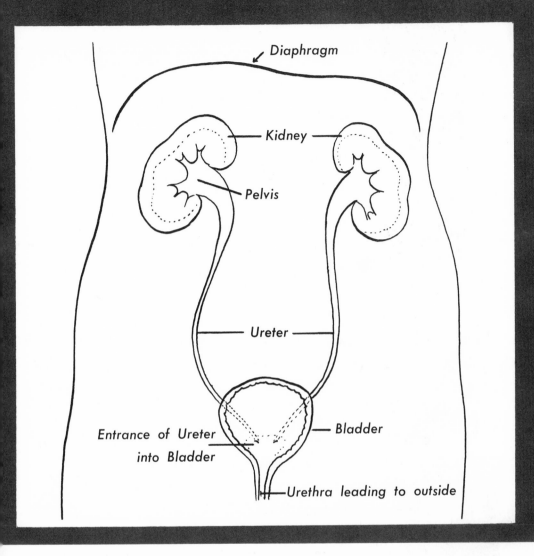

Normal Kidneys and Ureters. The kidneys manufacture urine, which is excreted down through the ureters and into the urinary bladder. Obstruction to the flow of urine down the ureters may cause severe damage to kidney substance and may eventually result in total loss of kidney function on the obstructed side.

What happens when kidney function is damaged?

   a. Excessive accumulation of chemical wastes and toxins in the bloodstream.

   b. Excessive loss of essential chemicals from the bloodstream into the urine.

   c. As a result of impaired kidney function, the tissues of the body are supplied with blood and solutions with improper chemical components. Eventually, if kidney function deteriorates beyond a certain point, such severe chemical upset occurs that life cannot continue.

Can one live a normal, healthy life with only one kidney?

Yes, provided the remaining kidney functions normally.

How can one tell if his kidney function is normal?

a. By analysis of the urine.

b. By chemical analysis of various constituents of the blood.

c. By x-ray examination of the kidneys and the rest of the urinary tract.

d. By special kidney function tests.

Is urine analysis always a good test for kidney diseases?

No. There are occasions when a kidney may be seriously damaged and yet the urine specimen may appear to be normal. However, by and large, urine analysis is a simple, rapid, and inexpensive initial test for screening.

What are the common causes of impaired kidney function?

a. Any generalized severe infection or inflammation.

b. Mechanical obstruction of the outlet of the kidneys.

c. General abnormalities of the kidneys which have existed since birth.

d. Tumors of the kidney.

e. Poisons which have been taken into the body and which damage kidney structure.

f. Interference with blood circulation to the kidneys.

g. Metabolic or hormone disease.

h. Abnormal concentrations of minerals in the bloodstream, or dehydration.

Is diabetes a kidney disease?

No. Diabetes is essentially a disease of the pancreas, but the

714

diagnosis is aided by examining the urine. (See Chapter 18, on Diabetes.)

Does swelling of the legs, the abdomen, and the face always indicate kidney disease?

Not necessarily. There are many other conditions which may cause this swelling.

Is it necessary to drink large quantities of water to make the kidneys function normally?

Let your thirst be your guide. This will usually provide sufficient fluid for adequate kidney function.

Are the advertised drugs which supposedly "flush the kidneys" beneficial?

No. Normal kidneys do their own flushing, and abnormal kidneys cannot be beneficially "flushed" by these drugs.

Do backaches usually indicate kidney disease?

The majority are not related to kidney disease. Certain types of backaches may be symptoms of a kidney disorder, but the diagnosis requires an examination by a physician.

What is the relationship between high blood pressure and kidney disease?

Long-standing high blood pressure over a period of years may eventually cause kidney disease due to disturbance in the circulation of the kidney. Conversely, severe kidney disorders often lead to high blood pressure.

Does albumin in the urine always indicate kidney disease?

Not necessarily. However, the presence of albumin must be considered to be indicative of a kidney disorder until further testing and procedures prove otherwise.

Does frequency of urination indicate kidney disease?

Sometimes, frequency of urination is caused merely by excessive drinking of fluids, or by nervous tension. On the other hand, disorders such as diabetes or enlargement of the prostate may be the cause of frequency of urination. Repeated episodes of frequency of urination should lead to a thorough investigation by your physician to rule out disturbance in kidney function.

Does bedwetting indicate kidney disease or a weak bladder?

No. Most cases have their origin in emotional disturbances.

Is salt restriction in the diet essential to a person with kidney disease?

Only in certain types of conditions.

Is water restriction advisable in chronic kidney disease?

Only in certain types of chronic kidney disease, namely, when undue amounts of fluid are already being retained by the body.

Can excessive eating of meats, eggs, or the intake of too much salt cause kidney disease?

No.

Does smoking hurt the kidneys?

No.

Is drinking of alcoholic beverages injurious to the kidneys?

Large quantities of alcohol may damage the kidneys, as it will all other tissues. It is well for a patient suffering from serious kidney disease not to drink alcoholic beverages.

Is the taking of large amounts of spices and condiments injurious to the kidneys?

Not usually. However, it can act as a temporary irritant when there already is disease in the urinary tract.

What is the significance of blood in the urine?

This should indicate that something is wrong somewhere in the urinary tract and the patient should seek medical advice promptly.

Does blood in the urine always indicate kidney disease?

No. The source of the blood may be the ureter, the bladder, or the urethra leading from the bladder to the outside.

Does cloudiness of the urine or pain on urination indicate kidney disease?

Not necessarily, although it may indicate that there is some disturbance within the urinary tract. Patients with such symptoms should seek medical advice promptly.

What is Bright's disease?

This is an old term, named after a famous physician, which denotes a variety of kidney diseases.

What is nephritis?

This is also a broad descriptive term denoting a diseased functioning of the kidneys.

GLOMERULONEPHRITIS

What is glomerulonephritis?

This is a specific disease which affects the nephrons of the kidney. It is caused by inflammation of the nephrons and may, if not checked, lead to scarring and destruction of these structures, with consequent impairment of kidney function.

What forms of glomerulonephritis are there?

a. Acute glomerulonephritis.
b. Chronic glomerulonephritis.

The acute stage may last from a few days to a year or more; the chronic stage may last as long as the patient lives. There is also an intermediate stage known as subacute glomerulonephritis.

How common a disease is acute glomerulonephritis?

It is quite a common condition, especially among children.

What causes acute glomerulonephritis?

Although the cause is not known, it usually appears shortly after a bacterial infection, most often after an infection caused by a streptococcus germ, which is commonly the cause of sore throats, tonsillitis, and scarlet fever.

What is the usual course of acute glomerulonephritis?

It usually lasts for several weeks and then subsides spontaneously. It is estimated that in children with acute glomerulonephritis, 75 to 90 per cent will get well without resultant kidney damage.

Is acute glomerulonephritis ever fatal?

Yes. In about one out of twenty cases, the patient may not survive this disease.

What are the symptoms of acute glomerulonephritis?

The patient may give a history of a previous acute infection, such as a severe sore throat. Blood and albumin may appear in the urine, with varying degrees of elevation of the blood pressure and tenderness over the kidney region.

At what age is acute glomerulonephritis most frequently seen?

Seventy per cent of all cases occur before the age of twenty-one.

Is nephritis of this type hereditary?

It is not thought to be hereditary, although there is a certain tendency for the condition to occur in families.

Is there any way to prevent getting nephritis?

All acute infections, especially sore throats, tonsillitis, and scarlet fever, should be treated promptly and thoroughly by a physician.

Is there any specific treatment for acute glomerulonephritis?

No. However, with proper rest and supportive measures, the majority of people will make a good recovery.

Is there any specific treatment for chronic glomerulonephritis?

No. However, people with chronic glomerulonephritis may live perfectly normal lives for many years if they take care of themselves by observing certain dietary precautions and avoiding acute infections.

NEPHROSIS

What is nephrosis?

It is a general term relating to certain types of kidney disorder in which there is generalized water-logging and swelling of the body tissues. This swelling and water-logging may be visible in the face, abdomen, and legs. There is also a loss of large quantities of body proteins, elevation of certain of the fatty substances in the blood-stream, and a lowering of the basal metabolism of the individual. There are many different specific causes of nephrosis.

Who is most likely to get nephrosis?

Children between the ages of two and seven years.

Is nephrosis a very common disease?

It is relatively rare.

What is the treatment for nephrosis?

This depends on the primary cause. General measures include diet and salt restrictions. Recently, cortisone and related chemicals have been used in certain types of cases with gratifying results.

Is it necessary to restrict salt intake in treating nephrosis?

Yes. Since retention of salt causes retention of water, it is important to restrict this substance.

Is restriction of meat, eggs, and other proteins recommended in nephrosis?

No.

What is the recovery rate from nephrosis?

In former years, about half the children with nephrosis would die. Today, with newer methods of treatment, three out of four will get well.

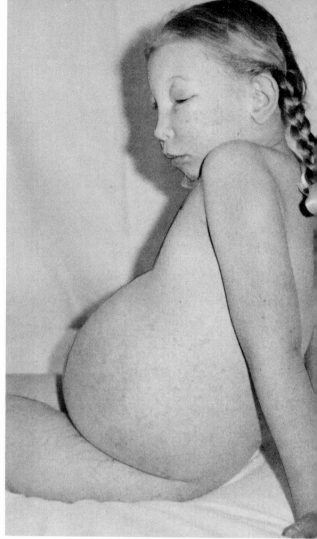

Nephrosis. This photograph shows an eight-year-old child with an advanced case of nephrosis. Fortunately, nephrotic children can now be helped greatly by the use of some of the newer drugs, such as cortisone, etc.

UREMIA

What is uremia?

This term denotes the abnormal chemical changes in the blood, as well as the associated symptoms, which appear in the advanced stages of kidney failure.

Can a patient with uremia recover?

Yes, provided that the cause is found and is capable of being eliminated. As an example, if it is caused by an obstruction of the ureter or the kidney outlet and this is promptly relieved, the uremia will subside and the patient will get well. If, on the other hand, it occurs in the end stages of a chronic nephritis, uremia is usually the terminal event ending in death.

PYELITIS AND PYELONEPHRITIS
(*Kidney Infections*)

What are pyelitis and pyelonephritis?

They are bacterial infections of the kidney, or the outlet of the kidney.

What causes pyelitis and pyelonephritis?

They are caused by bacteria which reach the kidney through the bloodstream, or by extension from other portions of the genito-urinary tract, such as the bladder, the prostate, the cervix, the vagina, or the urethra.

Who is most likely to develop pyelitis or pyelonephritis?

Pyelitis is seen quite often in children as an acute infection, but is also quite common in adults. Females, especially pregnant women, are more likely to develop kidney infection, since they are more prone to develop bladder infections. Also prone are diabetics and people who are debilitated or who have certain neurological disorders.

What are the symptoms of pyelitis or pyelonephritis?

High temperature, possibly with intermittent chills, backache, tenderness over the kidney area, frequency of urination along with painful voiding and blood in the urine. Nausea, vomiting, and lack of appetite are common. Examination may reveal pus and bacteria in the urine and an elevated white blood cell count.

Are both kidneys usually affected at the same time?

No, but this can occur in some cases.

What is the treatment for kidney infections?

   a. Drinking large quantities of fluids so as to flush out the pelvis and ureters of the kidneys.

b. Antibiotics to take care of the infecting organism.

c. Bed rest and a bland diet.

d. Medications for relief of pain.

What is the usual course of kidney infections?

Almost all patients get well. It is important to discover whether there is an underlying obstruction of the ureter which might have caused the urine to dam up and become infected, and it is important to eradicate any infection elsewhere in the body which might have precipitated the kidney infection.

How long is one usually ill with these infections?

Anywhere from a few days to several weeks.

Do antibiotics always prove effective in curing pyelitis or pyelonephritis?

In almost all instances, provided that the correct antibiotic drug is found for the particular bacteria causing the infection, and provided that other urinary tract defects are corrected.

Is hospitalization necessary in kidney infections?

The average case can be treated well at home. However, if the temperature is very high or if the pelvis of the kidney does not drain out its infected urine, then hospitalization is advisable.

What special hospital treatments may become necessary if the case does not respond to ordinary treatment?

The urologist may be called upon to pass a catheter (long rubber tube) into the bladder and then up into the ureter in order to drain out any infected urine which may be blocked in the pelvis of the kidney.

Is surgery necessary for pyelitis or pyelonephritis?

Usually not. However, if an abscess forms in or around the kidney, operative drainage may be necessary. Similarly, if the kidney infection is secondary to some other kidney disease, such as stones, surgery may be required.

Do kidney infections have a tendency to recur?

Yes, if there was a delay in the treatment of the initial attack or if treatment was inadequate. In these cases, lasting damage to the kidney occurs which may permanently impair its function.

Will frequent follow-up visits to a physician aid in preventing recurrence of kidney infection?

Yes.

Is it true that people with diabetes or heart disease are more prone to develop kidney infections?

Yes.

Does chronic kidney infection lead to the development of other diseases?

Yes. People with this condition often form stones, develop high blood pressure, and may eventually develop uremia.

KIDNEY STONES

What is the composition of kidney stones?

They are a combination of inorganic salts, such as calcium, phosphorus, ammonium, etc. They actually resemble the real stones which are present in the world of nature.

What causes the formation of kidney stones?

The exact mechanism is not known, but there are many theories:

a. Improper diet.
b. Chemical imbalance in the urine.
c. Disease of certain of the endocrine glands, such as the parathyroids.
d. Vitamin deficiencies.
e. Infection within the kidney.
f. Poor drainage in one or more parts of the urinary tract.

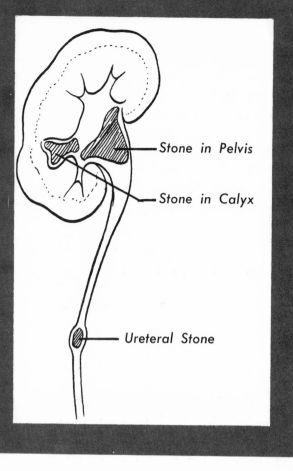

Stone in Pelvis

Stone in Calyx

Ureteral Stone

Kidney and Ureter Stones. This diagram shows kidney stones located in the pelvis of the kidney and in the ureters leading from the kidney. Such stones should be removed surgically. Operations for the removal of stones are safe and recovery takes place in almost all cases. If the stones have been causing obstruction for a long time, they may have produced permanent damage to kidney function.

Do kidney stones appear as frequently in both sexes?

No. They are somewhat more common in men.

Do kidney stones occur at any age?

Yes, but they are much more common in adults during the fourth, fifth, and sixth decades of life. Children do not get kidney stones very frequently.

What symptoms are caused by kidney stones?

In some instances the stones are quiescent and cause no symptoms. This type may be discovered accidentally. Usually, they do cause pain, blood and pus cells in the urine, and, not infrequently, they impair kidney function.

Do kidney stones tend to be single or multiple?

They are more often single but they may be multiple. When multiple stones are encountered, they may be found in both kidneys.

Is there much variation in the size of a kidney stone?

Yes. They vary in size from tiny fragments like grains of sand to stones that form an outline or cast of an entire kidney (staghorn or coral stones).

Must all kidney stones be removed surgically?

No. Many of them will pass spontaneously. Some are quiescent, cause no pain, no infection, and no interference with kidney function. The latter may be left alone. The stones that should be removed are those that appear to be too large to pass, those that cause obstruction and infection, those that cause constant pain or periodic attacks of severe pain, and those that appear to be causing progressive damage to kidney function.

Are there any *medications* which can be taken to dissolve kidney stones?

No! There are some dietary programs, such as low-phosphorus diet, an alkaline ash diet, or an acid diet, which may help to retard the growth of a stone or may help to prevent new stones from forming. There are also some drugs which have somewhat the same effect (Basalgel, acid salts, alkaline salts, etc.).

Are there any *solutions* which can be used to dissolve stones?

There are solutions which are helpful in reducing the size of stones, and in some cases actually dissolve them. However, these solutions must be brought into direct contact with the stone for a sufficient length of time to permit this to take place.

This means that if the stone is in the kidney, catheters must be put up to the kidney and left there for several days. This form of treatment is not universally applicable and cannot be used as a standard method.

Do kidney stones ever recur after they are once removed or passed?

Yes. However, dietary regulation, large fluid intake, the use of certain drugs, and the elimination of infection and obstruction of the urinary tract help to prevent their re-forming. Despite all precautions, in a small percentage of cases, stones will form again.

What are stones in the ureter?

The ureter is the tubelike structure connecting the kidney with the bladder. Stones rarely form primarily in the ureter, but kidney stones often pass down into the ureter and lodge there. When discovered there, they are known as ureteral stones.

What symptoms accompany stones in the ureter?

The principle symptom is excruciating pain of a colicky type. This may be so severe as to defy the effect of the most powerful narcotic drug. If the stone causes blockage of the flow of urine from the kidney, fever may result. If the urine is infected, the fever may be very high and may be accompanied by severe chills. Nausea, vomiting, and constipation are also common symptoms. Urinary discomfort, urgency, and frequency may be present. Blood in the urine is found in most cases.

What is the treatment for ureteral stones?

First, the pain must be controlled; next, if infection is present, it must be treated by the use of the antibiotic or sulfa drugs. If pain and infection cannot be controlled adequately, drainage of the kidney must be performed. This is done by passing a catheter beyond the stone through a cystoscope. If the catheter cannot be passed beyond the stone, then the stone must be removed surgically.

Is surgery usually necessary in the treatment of stones in the ureter?

No. Most stones in this location will pass spontaneously. If no infection supervenes, if the pain does not recur, and if the flow of urine is not blocked, then it is advisable to await the spontaneous passage of the stone. This may happen at any time within a period of several days or weeks.

When is surgery required for a ureter stone?

a. When the stone is obviously too large to pass.
b. If there is prolonged obstruction of urine.
c. If there are recurrent attacks of severe pain.
d. If infection persists.
e. If kidney function becomes impaired.

Can a stone ever be grasped by an instrument passed through a cysto-scope?

Yes. There are stone-grasping instruments which are sometimes successful in bringing a stone down through the ureter. If all of these methods fail, then surgery must be instituted.

Is the surgical removal of a stone in the ureter a serious operation?

It is a major procedure but carries with it virtually no mortality.

How long is the usual hospitalization period after surgery for a ureter stone?

Ten to twelve days.

Will the patient be able to live a completely normal life after surgery for a kidney stone?

Yes.

Should a patient who once had a kidney stone be checked periodically by his physician?

Yes. He should also follow all of the precautions mentioned previously to prevent re-formation of stones.

KIDNEY TUMORS

Who is most likely to get a tumor of the kidney?

Tumors of the kidney occur at any age, in either sex. However, the majority occur after the age of forty. One special type, called Wilm's tumor, occurs in infancy and childhood.

Are all kidney tumors malignant?

No, but the malignant tumors are seen more often than the benign ones.

What is the technical name for the most common malignant kidney tumor?

The most common kidney tumor is a hypernephroma.

How can one diagnose positively the presence of a kidney tumor?

By physical examination and by special x-rays of the kidneys, known as pyelograms.

What is an intravenous pyelogram?

It is an x-ray procedure in which a radio-opaque solution is injected into the bloodstream. The solution is excreted by the kidneys, and as it is being excreted it outlines the kidneys, which are visualized by taking an x-ray.

Is an intravenous pyelogram a painful or dangerous procedure?

No. However, if the patient is markedly allergic, special precautions must be taken before this procedure is carried out.

Are pyelograms important in making a diagnosis in other kidney diseases besides tumors?

Yes. It will show the presence of many other abnormalities within the urinary tract. It is also valuable in making a diagnosis of prostate enlargement or the presence of stones in the prostate gland.

What symptoms and signs do kidney tumors produce?
   a. Blood in the urine.
   b. Pain in the loin over the kidney region.
   c. The presence of a mass or lump in the kidney area.

What is the treatment for a kidney tumor?

Prompt removal of the entire kidney. Preliminary x-ray therapy and postoperative x-ray treatments are also advised in certain types of kidney tumor.

Is the removal of a kidney a serious operation?

Yes, but if the opposite kidney is normal, the removal of one kidney will not adversely affect life.

Right: X-ray Showing Outlines of Normal Kidneys and Ureters. These outlines are obtained by injecting a dye substance into the veins and taking x-rays at the time the dye reaches the kidneys.

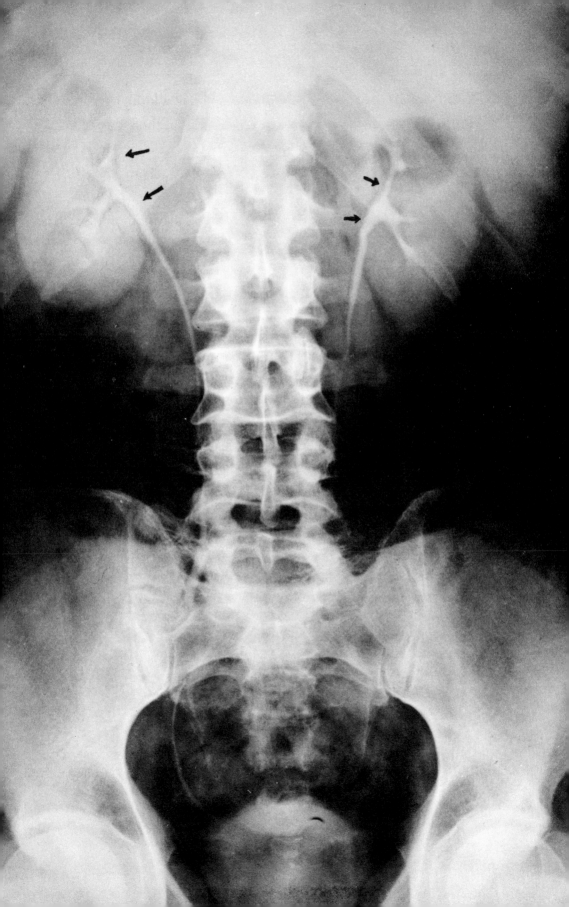

Is kidney removal (nephrectomy) a dangerous operation?

No. Recovery, with an uncomplicated postoperative course, is the usual outcome.

How long is the patient in the hospital after an operation for removal of a kidney?

Ten to twelve days.

CYSTS OF THE KIDNEY

What are some of the common forms of cystic disease of the kidney?

a. Congenital polycystic kidneys. This is a condition with which one is born and is characterized by numerous large and small cysts, usually of both kidneys. Kidney function is impaired in this type of disease as the individual grows older.

b. Solitary cyst of the kidney. This type usually does not impair kidney function.

What are the symptoms in polycystic kidney disease?

As the patient grows into adulthood there may be pain in the kidney area, blood in the urine, infection, and elevated blood pressure.

What are the symptoms of solitary cyst of the kidney?

Usually, there are no symptoms. Occasionally, there may be pain and blood in the urine.

What is the treatment for polycystic kidneys?

There is no effective treatment for the cysts themselves. When complications arise, such as infection, stone formation or excessive pain, these are treated by ordinary measures.

What is the treatment for a solitary cyst of the kidney?

The cyst itself is removed, leaving the remainder of the kidney in place. Once in a great while, a solitary cyst can be treated by withdrawing the fluid and injecting a solution which induces the cyst to close itself off. This is not, however, the most common method of handling solitary cysts.

CONGENITAL DEFECTS OF THE KIDNEY
(Birth Abnormalities)

Is the kidney subject to many types of congenital abnormalities?

Yes. There may be only one kidney instead of two; there may be one or two small additional kidneys; the kidneys may be in the wrong position in the body (ectopic kidneys); both kidneys may be on the same side of the body; the kidneys may be joined across the midline of the body (horseshoe kidney); the collecting portions of the kidney (pelvis) may be duplicated; the ureters may be duplicated.

An important abnormality is the presence of a narrowing or stricture at the kidney pelvis at the junction between the kidney and ureter. Such a condition may impede the normal flow of urine and eventually lead to obstruction of the kidney and impairment of its function.

Do most congenital abnormalities of the kidneys cause symptoms?

No, with the exception of the strictures which cause the symptoms listed above.

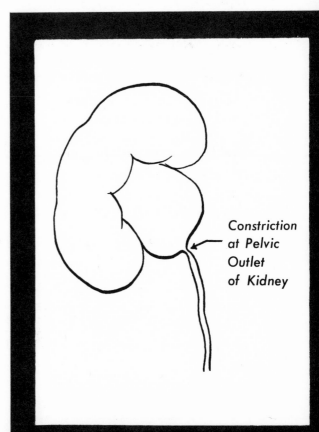

Constriction
at Pelvic
Outlet
of Kidney

Constriction at the Outlet of the Kidney. Such a condition often requires surgical reconstruction to relieve the obstruction to the flow of urine.

Are these abnormal kidneys more prone to infection?

Yes.

What is the treatment for the congenital obstruction at the junction between the kidney and the ureter?

Where there is advanced obstruction of the kidney or where the kidney function is impaired, surgery is indicated.

What surgery is carried out for obstruction of the kidney at its junction with the ureter?

A plastic operation is performed to widen the passageway, or simple attempts to dilate the stricture with dilating instruments may be made in some cases.

Are operations for obstruction at the kidney outlet serious?

Yes, but they are not dangerous. They do involve a long hospitalization, usually three to four weeks, and the patient may have to carry tubes which are inserted to splint and drain the area while healing takes place.

Are the results of these operations successful?

Yes, in the great majority of cases.

KIDNEY INJURIES

What are the common causes for kidney injuries?

a. Automobile accidents.

b. Athletic events, such as football or boxing.

c. A fall from a height with a direct blow to the kidney area.

How can one tell if he has a kidney injury?

a. By noting pain and tenderness in the kidney region.

b. By noting blood in the urine.

What is the treatment for kidney injuries?

For the minor injuries, which make up the great majority, bed rest is the main form of treatment. If the bleeding is alarming and the x-ray shows a badly damaged kidney, surgery may become necessary for removal of the organ.

Can a damaged kidney ever be restored surgically?

Yes. If the damage has not been too extensive, the kidney may be sutured instead of being removed.

Is it often necessary to operate for a kidney injury?

The great majority will get well without surgery.

How can one tell whether surgery is necessary?

By noting whether the urine clears and whether there is evidence of restored kidney function. If blood continues to appear in the urine and kidney function fails to return, surgery is indicated.

TUBERCULOSIS OF THE KIDNEYS
(See Chapter 68, on Tuberculosis.)

Is tuberculosis of the kidneys often a primary disease?

No. It is usually secondary to tuberculosis of the lungs.

How does tuberculosis reach the kidneys?

The germs are carried to it through the bloodstream.

What are the symptoms of kidney tuberculosis?

Frequent, painful urination and bloody urine.

How is the diagnosis of tuberculosis of the kidney made?

By finding the tuberculosis germs in the urine. It is often necessary to inoculate animals (guinea pigs) with the urine to see whether they develop tuberculosis several weeks later. There are also characteristic x-ray findings which help to make the diagnosis. When tuberculosis has involved the bladder, cystoscopic examination will reveal a characteristic appearance.

What is the treatment for tuberculosis of the kidney?

In the early stages, the disease may be arrested with the use of some of the newer anti-tuberculosis drugs. If the disease is limited to one kidney and has already produced marked destruction, the use of drugs *and* surgical removal of the kidney may be indicated. Where both kidneys are involved, drug treatment is preferable. The drugs used are streptomycin, isoniazid, and para-amino-salicylic acid.

If tuberculosis is limited to one kidney and that kidney is removed, can a cure be obtained?

We do not speak of cures in tuberculosis, but rather of *arrest* of the disease. If the disease is limited to one kidney, its removal will arrest the disease.

"DROPPED KIDNEY" OR "FLOATING KIDNEY"
(Nephroptosis)

What is a dropped or floating kidney?

A kidney which has become detached from its moorings and drops to an abnormally low position in the body.

What type of person is most likely to have a floating kidney?

Thin individuals, especially women.

Is a dropped kidney more likely to be seen on the right side?

Yes.

What are the symptoms of a dropped kidney?

If any symptoms are present, they will consist of backache and abdominal pain. The kinking of the outlet of the kidney may interfere with the ready outflow of urine. This may result in a so-called "renal crisis," with attacks of severe colicky pain in the kidney area.

Is it necessary to treat a dropped kidney which causes no symptoms?

No.

Dropped Kidney. In certain people, a kink develops in a ureter associated with a dropped kidney and this will cause marked pain in the loin. People who are very thin or who have lost large amounts of weight are especially subject to this condition. Symptoms often improve when the patient gains weight. In other cases, it is necessary to operate to tack down the kidney in a more normal position.

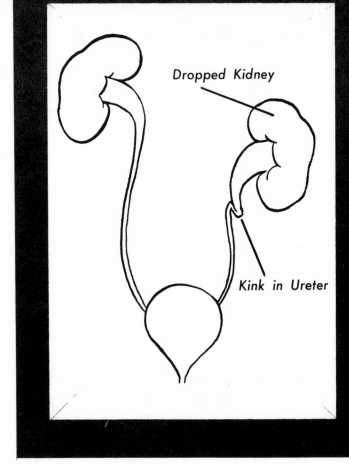

Dropped Kidney

Kink in Ureter

What treatment is indicated when the dropped kidney does cause symptoms?

    a. Medical management, with a special diet to increase body weight and the wearing of a support or corset to keep the kidney in its proper position.

    b. A surgical procedure in which the kidney is fixed by sutures into its normal position. Such an operation is called a nephropexy.

Are operations for a dropped kidney serious?

    No. The results are good. Hospitalization for a period of ten to twelve days is usually necessary.

Are blood transfusions usually necessary when performing major kidney surgery?

    Yes.

Should private nurses be engaged when kidney surgery is performed?
Yes, for a period of two to three days.

How long a convalescent period is required after kidney operations?
Approximately one month.

TUMORS OF THE URETER

Are tumors of the ureter very common?
No. They are extremely rare.

What forms do tumors of the ureter usually take?
The great majority of them are malignant.

What are the symptoms of tumors of the ureter?
Blood in the urine, obstruction to the passage of urine into the bladder, and eventual infection.

How is the diagnosis of a tumor of the ureter made?
By x-ray studies of the urinary tract and by noting obstruction on attempted passage of a catheter up the ureter.

What is the treatment for a tumor of the ureter?
Removal of the ureter along with its kidney and a portion of the bladder surrounding the entrance of the ureter.

Are operations of this type serious?
Yes, but recovery can be expected in the great majority of cases.

Can tumors of the ureter be cured by surgery?
Yes, when they are discovered at an early stage and when the operation, as outlined above, is carried out.

How long a hospital stay is necessary after operations of this type?
Approximately two to three weeks.

URETEROCELE

What is a ureterocele?

A cystic formation at the bladder end of the ureter due to an abnormal opening of the ureter into the bladder. There is also a weakness in the wall of the ureter in its lowermost portion, probably the result of a birth deformity.

What are the symptoms of a ureterocele?

There may be no symptoms at all and the condition may be discovered accidentally during the course of a routine investigation for some other condition in the urinary tract. Ureteroceles can, however, be the cause of a chronic infection in the bladder and kidney.

What is the treatment for a ureterocele?

If it is a small one, it can be treated successfully by enlarging the opening of the ureter into the bladder. Some ureteroceles may be treated through a cystoscope, either by burning off a portion of the cyst or by shaving off a portion of it. If the ureterocele is large, it may be necessary to operate and remove it through an opening made in the bladder.

Are operations for ureterocele successful?

Yes.

Are these operations dangerous?

No.

Laboratory (Pathology) Tests, Procedures, and Treatments

34

What is a pathologist?

A physician who specializes in laboratory medicine and who works closely with other physicians as a consultant in the diagnosis and treatment of disease.

What are the usual duties of a pathologist?

To interpret laboratory tests performed upon patients, to examine human tissues which have been removed from patients, and to determine the cause of death in certain cases by making autopsy examinations. He may also render certain specific treatments, such as the giving of intravenous infusions or blood transfusions.

In addition to the above duties, is the pathologist responsible for the operation of a clinical and pathologic laboratory?

Yes.

What types of tests do these laboratories usually perform?

a. All types of blood tests.

b. Urine analysis.

c. Stool analysis.

d. Sputum analysis.

e. Analysis of the stomach and duodenal contents (gastric analysis).

   f. Bone marrow analysis.

   g. Blood chemistries.

   h. Blood cultures for circulating bacteria.

   i. Pus cultures.

   j. Spinal fluid examinations.

   k. Examination of fluid or material from various other cavities of the body, such as in lung taps or abdominal taps.

   l. Pregnancy tests, and other endocrine tests.

   m. Animal inoculations to discover the cause for disease.

What treatments are often carried out by pathologists in their laboratories?

   a. The giving of blood transfusions.

   b. The giving of other substances into the veins or beneath the skin.

Taking Blood for a Blood Count. This procedure is almost painless, and the information to be gained from the blood count is very important. People should have a complete blood count performed whenever they have been ill for a period of several weeks or more.

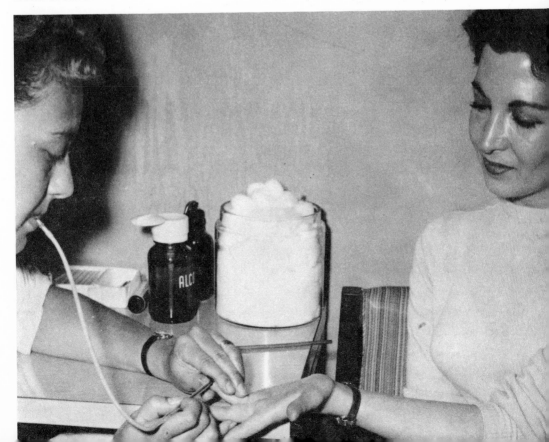

c. The manufacture and administration of specially prepared vaccines.

d. The handling of special problems relating to blood diseases and to bleeding tendencies.

Why is it necessary for a patient to make a special appointment before going to a laboratory for a test or series of tests?

Appointments are advisable because it is often necessary for the patient to make special preparations, such as not eating for a certain number of hours before coming to the laboratory. Many tests cannot be carried out unless special instructions are given beforehand as to how to prepare for them.

Is it usually best to have blood tests performed upon a fasting stomach?

Yes, especially for those blood tests concerned with the chemistry

This picture shows a laboratory technician performing a blood count and examining a smear of the blood under the microscope. Blood diseases such as anemia and many others can be definitely determined by examining the drop of blood removed from the fingertip.

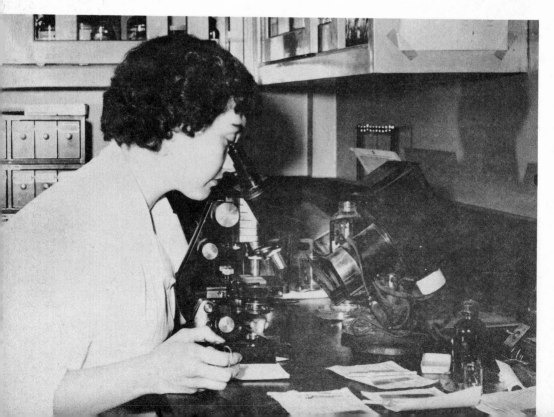

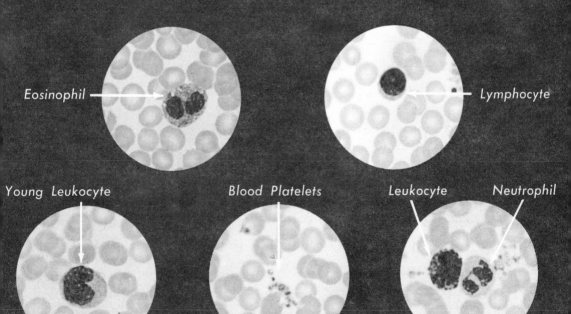

Monocyte

Eosinophil

Lymphocyte

Young Leukocyte

Blood Platelets

Leukocyte

Neutrophil

Blood Smear. This photomicrograph shows what red blood cells look like under the microscope. Variations in the size, shape, and number of blood cells are frequently diagnostic of specific diseases, and the pathologist also learns a great deal about all aspects of the patient's health merely by examining a sample of blood under the microscope.

of the blood. In those instances, a twelve-hour period of fasting should precede the test.

BLOOD TESTS

What is a complete blood count, and how is it taken?

This is a test performed by pricking the finger or the lobe of the ear. It can be taken at any time without special preparation. A complete blood count will show whether or not the patient has anemia or whether or not the body is suffering from any generalized infection.

Is it painful when the vein is punctured for a blood test?

There is only very slight pain if a good sharp needle is used.

How does the taking of a blood count show anemia?

By counting the number of red blood cells, noting the amount of hemoglobin in the cells, and noting the characteristic appearance of the blood under the microscope.

Can a pathologist diagnose the varying types of anemia by examination of the blood?

Yes. There are many types of anemia and the treatment for each may be different.

How does a blood count indicate infection?

By an increase in the white blood cell count and by a characteristic shift of the type of white blood cell which appears when there is an acute infection.

Is the taking of a white blood count frequently important in determining the seriousness of the illness and in determining whether or not an operation is necessary, such as in the case of a possible appendicitis?

Yes. This is a most valuable test in helping to make a decision.

What is hemoglobin?

The iron-containing pigment in red blood cells which carries oxygen to the cells throughout the body.

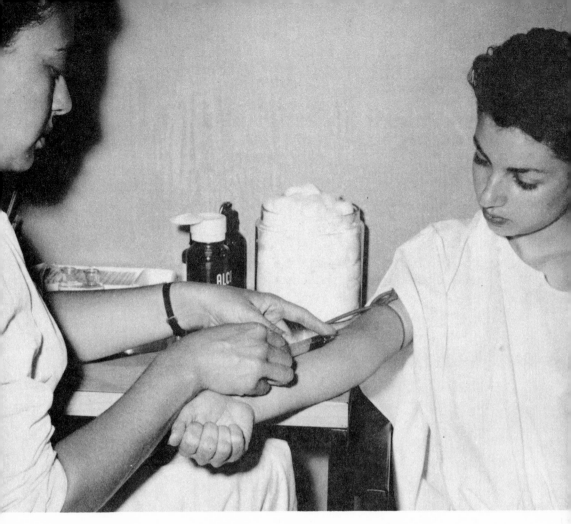

Vein Puncture. Patient having blood removed from vein in arm. The main reason for withdrawing blood from a vein is to analyze it for chemical constituents. Many diseases can be diagnosed by noting abnormalities in the chemical components of blood. There is only slight pain when the vein is punctured.

Why is it necessary to have a blood test before tonsils are removed?

The tendency of the tissues to bleed and the blood to clot should be recorded before tonsils are removed. When these tests, known as bleeding time and clotting time, are normal, the surgeon can proceed without fear of hemorrhage due to an abnormal condition of the blood.

Can anemia be successfully treated by blood transfusions?

Blood transfusions may temporarily correct the deficiency, but they do not relieve the underlying cause of the anemia and therefore cannot produce a permanent cure. There is one exception, and that is when anemia has been caused solely by sudden hemorrhage. In this instance blood transfusion can bring about a cure of the anemia.

Can the taking of a blood count determine whether a child has lead poisoning?

Up to a certain point, yes. In microscopic examination, the red blood cells usually show anemia and a characteristic stippled appearance. This disease was quite prevalent in the days when toys were coated with paint containing lead. The child would chew on the toys and develop lead poisoning. Even today, painters who use leaded paints in their work are subject to this disease.

What is a heterophile antibody test?

This is a test useful in the diagnosis of infectious mononucleosis.

What is a sedimentation rate?

This is a test performed after drawing a small amount of blood from a vein in the arm. The withdrawn blood is placed in a special glass tube containing an anticoagulant, and the blood cells are allowed to separate out from the plasma. The rate at which the blood cells drop to the bottom of the tube is called the sedimentation rate. It is a rough index of the presence or absence of inflammation somewhere in the body. The more rapid the sedimentation rate, the more likely that an inflammatory process exists.

When is a sedimentation rate most likely to be recommended by the physician?

In certain cases of pelvic inflammation in women, or when the blood count itself does not give all the information that is desired. If the blood sediments rapidly, it is usually an indication that inflammation or infection is present.

What is a Wassermann or serology test?

It is a test to determine the presence or absence of syphilis. A negative Wassermann test usually denotes the absence of syphilis. However, a positive Wassermann does not necessarily mean that the patient has syphilis.

Are there any other blood tests to determine the absence or presence of syphilis?

Yes. There are many modifications of the Wassermann test, but their general purpose and results are about the same.

What is a dark-field examination?

This is a test whereby material is taken from an ulcer or other lesion suspected as being syphilitic and examined directly under a special microscope. The finding of typical spirochetes is diagnostic. The test should be performed only by individuals who have special training and experience in the technique.

Is the diagnosis of syphilis made from the blood test alone?

Never. The clinical history, physical examination, and findings are just as important as the results of the blood test.

What is a bone marrow study?

A test in which a small amount of marrow is obtained from the breastbone or some other bone by placing a needle into it. It enables the physician to see how well the blood is being formed and whether it contains tissues or cells which should not normally be present.

Is a bone marrow test painful?

There is only very slight pain, since a local anesthetic is used before the needle is inserted.

Is a bone marrow study important in determining the presence or absence of blood diseases and various types of anemia?

Yes. It is an extremely valuable test and should always be done whenever there is doubt as to the exact diagnosis.

Who should perform a blood marrow test?

The pathologist or other specialist qualified in the diagnosis of diseases of the blood.

BLOOD TRANSFUSIONS

When are blood transfusions most valuable?

a. When there has been an acute, sudden loss of blood due to disease or injury.

b. When an acute loss of blood is anticipated, such as when a major operation is to be performed.

c. To give the patient a temporary lift until his own bone marrow can resume the manufacture of blood, as after a prolonged or debilitating disease which has produced anemia.

Should blood transfusions be given under the direct supervision of a physician?

Yes, most emphatically. A transfusion means taking blood from a healthy individual and injecting it into a patient. This is a serious procedure and is sometimes associated with complications demanding expert knowledge.

Who should perform the blood grouping (typing), preparatory to the giving of a blood transfusion?

A well-qualified laboratory employing expert technicians should always be used to type the patient's blood. Accidents occur if correct typing and cross-matching are not performed.

What complications can occur from giving the wrong type of blood?

Chills and fever, jaundice, or even death may ensue from giving improperly cross-matched blood.

Should people know their blood groups (types), so that if an accident should occur they can be transfused more quickly?

Yes. It is wise to know one's own blood group. The blood must always be re-examined prior to transfusion. The blood to be given must always be matched with the recipient's blood before transfusion.

When given under proper supervision, are blood transfusions safe?

Yes.

Patient Receiving a Blood Transfusion. The bottle at the side of the bed contains blood. (Most of it has already dripped into the patient's vein.) Blood is obtained from donors and is stored in the laboratory until needed. It is essential that the blood grouping of the donor be the same as that of the recipient. Such cross-matching of bloods is carried out in the laboratory before the transfusion is given.

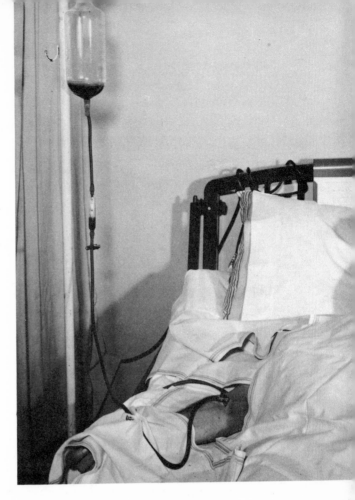

What are some of the complications of blood transfusions?

   a. Chills and fever. This is a common complication.

   b. Allergic reactions, such as hives, asthma, etc. When this occurs, the transfusion is usually stopped.

   c. Jaundice. This may occur as long as three to four months after the transfusion has been given.

   d. Shock, from giving the wrong type of blood or contaminated blood. This is an extremely rare event.

Can infants and children be given transfusions?

   Yes.

Are there satisfactory methods for combating reactions to transfusions?

   Yes. Most reactions can be mitigated by proper medical treatment.

What is meant by an "exchange transfusion"?

This is a special type of blood transfusion usually performed on new-borns who have a blood condition known as erythroblastosis. It attempts to exchange all or most of the infant's blood for new blood and thus get rid of the blood causing the disease. This must be performed only by an expert in the field.

What is a blood bank?

There are special blood laboratories set up in large hospitals and institutions where blood is collected from donors and is stored. Blood may be kept for periods up to three weeks prior to use. It is an excellent idea, because the bank tries to maintain a supply of blood of all types to meet any emergency.

BLOOD CHEMISTRY

What is a blood chemistry?

It is a test performed on venous blood to determine the amount of the various minerals and chemicals circulating in the body.

What are some of the usual chemicals and minerals tested for when a blood chemistry is taken?

a. Albumin.
b. Calcium.
c. Carbon dioxide content.
d. Chloride.
e. Cholesterol.
f. Creatinine.
g. Globulin.
h. Icterus index.
i. Non-protein nitrogen.

j. Phospatase.
k. Phosphorus.
l. Potassium.
m. Sodium.
n. Sugar.
o. Total protein.
p. Urea nitrogen.
q. Uric acid.

Are blood chemistries valuable in diagnosing the presence or absence of disease?

Yes. In certain instances, the diagnosis cannot be made without a characteristic blood test.

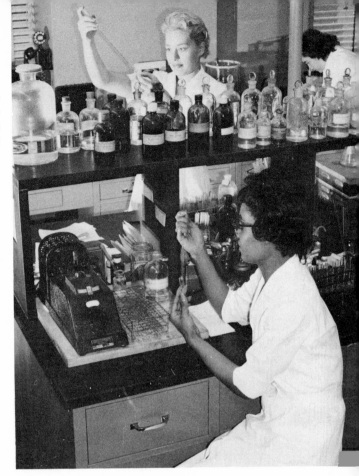

Laboratory technicians performing chemical analysis upon a specimen of blood. It usually takes two to three days before chemical analysis of blood is completed.

What are some of the diseases which are revealed by characteristic changes in the blood chemistry or blood tests?

a. Diabetes mellitus.

b. Nephritis.

c. Uremia.

d. Gout.

e. Certain bone diseases.

f. Certain types of jaundice.

g. Certain liver diseases.

h. Many other serious illnesses.

Are characteristic findings in the blood chemistry helpful in determining treatment for disease?

Yes. The quantity of a certain chemical circulating in the blood is often an essential factor in deciding what form of treatment should be given.

Does life ever depend upon the amount of certain chemicals circulating in the blood?

Definitely, yes. An excessive amount of certain chemicals or an excessive lack of certain chemicals may throw the patient into shock, coma, and may eventually lead to death.

Can blood chemicals be artificially replaced?

Yes. One of the most common forms of treatment for serious disease is to have certain of the chemicals, which may be lacking, given by mouth or by injecting them under the skin or directly into the bloodstream.

GLUCOSE TOLERANCE TEST

What is a glucose tolerance test?

A test in which the fasting patient is given a known amount of glucose (sugar) by mouth and the blood is tested at intervals thereafter to note the quantity of sugar in the blood. A curve is then constructed from which important information can be drawn.

What will a glucose tolerance test curve show?

a. Whether the patient is a diabetic.
b. Whether the patient has too little sugar in his blood (hyperinsulinism).
c. Characteristic changes in certain other hormonal disturbances.

Will blood tests in diabetic patients usually show an excessive amount of sugar?

Yes.

BLOOD CULTURES

Of what value are blood cultures?

In diseases in which one suspects that bacteria are circulating in the bloodstream, blood is taken to the laboratory and is cultured to see if bacteria will grow from the blood.

What types of diseases may show positive blood cultures?

Cases of blood poisoning (septicemia).

Are blood tests valuable in determining the various types of jaundice?

Yes. A distinction can usually be made between obstructive jaundice which is due to the prevention of outflow of bile from the liver, jaundice which is due to an inflammation or disease within the liver, and jaundice which is due to an excessive destruction of blood.

Are blood tests valuable in diagnosing the quantity of cholesterol which is in the blood?

Yes. It is now a matter of a great deal of medical thought because some investigators feel that hardening of the arteries is associated with an excessive amount of cholesterol in the body.

Are there any blood tests which will give information about metabolism?

Yes. The determination of protein-bound iodine in the blood is one such test. It is even more accurate than the basal metabolism rate in determining the state of underactivity or overactivity of the thyroid gland.

URINE ANALYSIS

Are drugstores sufficiently well equipped to perform urine analysis?

No. Whenever possible, a well-qualified pathology laboratory should be used to carry out urine analyses. These are very important tests and should not be entrusted to improperly equipped laboratories.

When is it usually best to collect one's urine for testing?

Most urines, except for certain special tests, should be collected in a clean bottle as the first specimen passed in the morning.

For what substances is the ordinary urine specimen tested?

a. Albumin.
b. Sugar.
c. Acidity or alkalinity.
d. Presence or absence of pus.
e. Presence or absence of blood cells, both red and white.
f. Presence or absence of bile pigment, as in cases of jaundice.

g. Presence or absence of casts (microscopic forms denoting kidney damage).

h. Presence or absence of crystals of certain chemicals.

What can be learned from the presence or absence of these substances in the urine?

Examination of urine gives valuable information concerning the state of health of the kidneys or other portions of the urinary tract. In addition, it may suggest the presence of diabetes, liver disease, etc.

Does the finding of abnormal substances in the urine always denote the presence of disease?

Not always. Sometimes these are transient findings. It is therefore important to repeat urine tests at regular intervals before making a diagnosis of disease.

Is it often wise to double-check findings on urine analysis by testing the blood?

Yes. Urine analysis is a helpful test but not always a conclusive one.

Are there any reliable chemical tests on urine or blood specific for cancer?

No.

PREGNANCY TESTS

Are pregnancy tests conducted on the urine?

Yes.

How accurate are pregnancy tests?

Most laboratories report about 95 per cent accuracy in their pregnancy tests.

Is it wise, if the examination by the physician does not seem to coincide with the pregnancy test, to repeat the test?

Yes. It is occasionally necessary to repeat the urine pregnancy test several times before coming to a definite conclusion.

How are pregnancy tests carried out?

By injecting the urine or its concentrate into suitable animals, such as mice, frogs, rabbits, etc. The reaction in the animal takes a variable length of time to develop.

How long does it take to get the result of a pregnancy test?

It varies with the different test animals. However, an answer can usually be given within two days.

How soon after a woman thinks she is pregnant would a pregnancy test show a conclusive result?

For utmost reliability, a woman should not have the test performed before the tenth day following the day of the first missed menstrual period.

Is the pregnancy test always positive if there is a pregnancy in the Fallopian tube?

No. The pregnancy test in tubal (ectopic) pregnancy is not nearly as important as the physical examination performed by the physician.

RH TEST

What is an Rh test?

An Rh test determines the presence or absence of the Rh factor in the blood. It is done whenever a person's blood is typed.

Should all pregnant women have Rh factor blood tests done upon them?

Definitely, yes.

Why is the Rh factor important in pregnancy?

It is particularly important in pregnancy because Rh negative women (those who lack the Rh factor), when married to men who are Rh positive, may carry an embryo which is Rh positive. These women may become sensitized to the Rh factor in the unborn child. Under ordinary circumstances, this does the mother no harm, but it may affect the baby.

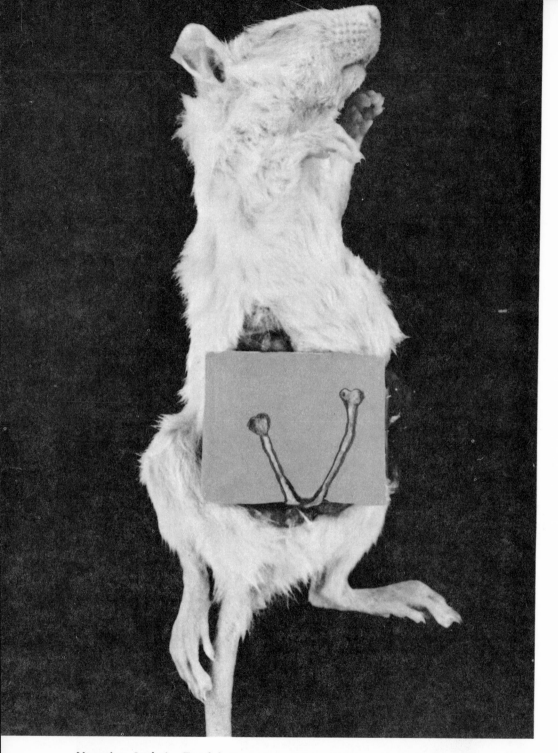

Negative Ascheim-Zondek Pregnancy Test. This is a photograph showing the tubes and ovaries of a mouse to be of normal size two days after the injection of a sample of urine from a patient. This response is negative, showing that the patient is not pregnant.

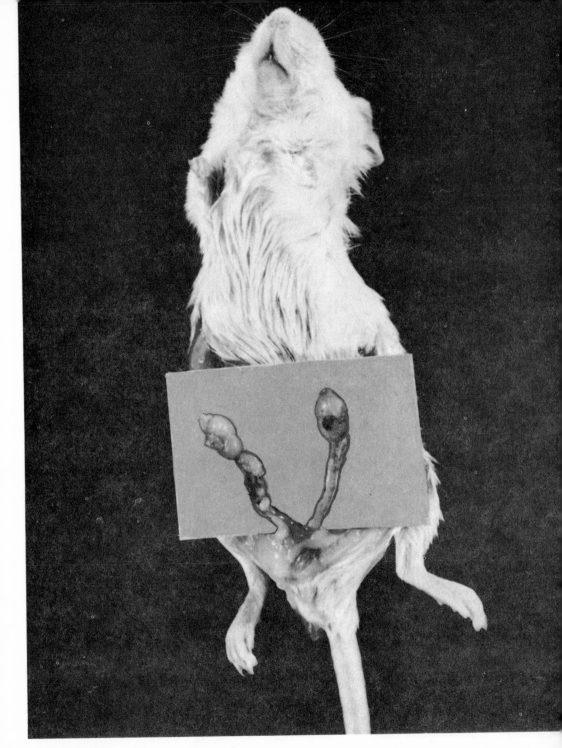

Positive Ascheim-Zondek Pregnancy Test. This shows markedly swollen tubes and ovaries, thus indicating a positive A-Z pregnancy test. It takes two to three days from the time of injection of these mice until the final reading of the tests. Such tests are accurate in more than 90 per cent of cases.

If a mother is Rh negative, will her baby require a blood transfusion?

The baby will require a transfusion only if the mother has been sensitized to the Rh factor and antibodies produced by the mother affect the baby. The fact that the mother is Rh negative does not, in itself mean that her baby will require any treatment at all.

What is erythroblastosis?

This is a condition in the newborn in which blood cells are destroyed in huge quantities because of difficulties with the Rh factor.

Is erythroblastosis a dangerous condition?

Yes. If not treated promptly, it may lead to death of the infant.

Should difficulty with the Rh factor influence a woman not to have more children?

In the great majority of cases, the Rh factor will not produce difficulties, and therefore women should not be fearful of having more children. However, each case must be carefully studied by a physician experienced in this field, and advice should be sought from him.

Is it possible for an Rh negative woman married to an Rh positive man to bear an Rh negative infant?

Yes.

Is it possible for an Rh positive woman to bear a child who will have complications due to other blood factors?

Yes. Other factors in the blood may at times cause trouble, but these are usually of far less importance and severity than the Rh factor.

How can one predict whether an unborn child will have trouble because of the Rh factor?

The mother's blood can be tested for anti-Rh antibodies during the course of her pregnancy. These afford a rough index of what may be expected when the baby is born.

What are antibody studies?

These are tests to determine whether the body has produced antibodies.

What is the danger of antibodies in a person sensitized to the Rh factor?

The antibodies have no effect on the person so sensitized unless they are transfused or get an injection of Rh positive blood. In this case, a severe reaction may develop.

Can a sensitized woman who remarries bear normal children?

Yes, if the new husband is Rh negative or of a blood group other than the one which caused the original sensitization.

Is there any difference between an erythroblastotic baby and a blue baby?

Yes. A blue baby is one who has a congenital disease of the heart or lungs. An erythroblastotic baby is one who suffers as a result of his mother's sensitization to the Rh factor in the blood.

Will an erythroblastotic baby be a normal baby if it survives?

If the damage to the baby incident to the disease is minimal, and this is usually the case, such a baby will almost always develop normally.

Is there any way of preventing the development of erythroblastosis in babies to be born of a mother known to have been sensitized to the Rh factor?

There are no injections or drugs known at present which will prevent the disease.

Can the first child of an Rh negative woman have erythroblastosis?

This is rare, but it can happen if she has previously been sensitized to the Rh factor by means of an injection or transfusion containing the Rh factor.

What is the treatment for erythroblastosis?

Exchange transfusion to replace the baby's Rh positive blood with the donor's Rh negative blood.

GASTRIC ANALYSIS

What is a gastric analysis?

A test whereby the secretions of the stomach are removed and the constituents are analyzed.

What is looked for in a gastric analysis?
a. The presence or absence of hydrochloric acid which should normally be secreted by the cells lining the stomach.
b. The presence or absence of lactic acid, a substance which should not normally be present in the stomach.
c. The presence or absence of blood which should not normally be present in the stomach.
d. The presence or absence of cancer cells which, by special tests, can be noted in the gastric secretions of those who have cancer of the stomach.

In what conditions are gastric analyses most important?
a. In pernicious anemia. In this condition an absence of hydrochloric acid is found.
b. In ulcer of the stomach or duodenum. In these conditions an excessive amount of acid is often found.
c. In tumors of the stomach. In such conditions, the presence of lactic acid or even the presence of actual cancer cells may be determined on analysis of the gastric content.
d. In tuberculosis, when it is suspected that sputum is being swallowed instead of being expectorated.

How is a gastric analysis performed?

By placing a rubber tube into the mouth or nose and passing it down into the stomach.

Is this a very painful test?

Not at all, although it is somewhat unpleasant.

How long does a gastric analysis take to perform?

This is determined by the purpose of the test. It may take only a few minutes or it may require three hours to complete.

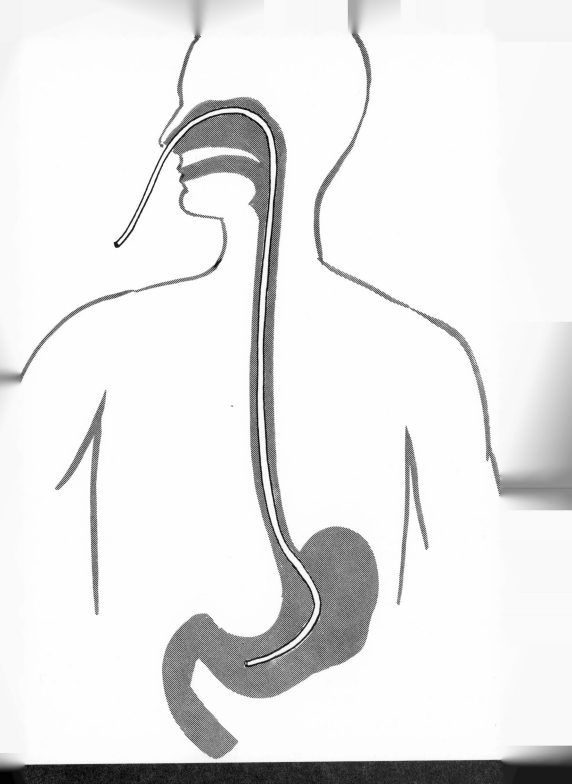

Gastric Analysis. This diagram shows a rubber tube which has been inserted through the nose, down the esophagus, and into the stomach in order to perform an analysis of the stomach contents. The contents are analyzed for acid, the presence or absence of blood, and other substances. Gastric analysis, while uncomfortable, is not a painful procedure; most people undergo it without complaint.

Must a gastric analysis be performed on a fasting stomach?

Yes.

Where are gastric analysis tests carried out?

Usually, in the office of a well-equipped laboratory. Also, the test is frequently performed upon hospitalized patients.

Is there any danger involved in having a gastric analysis test performed?

None whatever.

PAPANICOLAOU TEST

What is a Papanicolaou smear?

This is a test whereby smears are taken from accessible organs, usually the vagina or uterine cervix in the female, for the diagnosis of cancer. It has a high degree of reliability in the hands of persons trained in performing this procedure. It should be noted that a negative result is of far less value than a positive one. The latter should be confirmed by additional examinations. (See Chapter 15 on Cancer.)

How is a Papanicolaou smear performed?

By taking a cotton swab or other instrument and scraping off the superficial cells from the vagina or from the cervix, and smearing the obtained material onto glass slides. These are then stained by a special technique and examined under the microscope.

Is this a painful or unpleasant test?

Not at all.

Who should take Papanicolaou smears?

The gynecologist, or other examining physician, in his office.

BIOPSY

What is a biopsy?

It is the removal of tissue by a physician or surgeon, who sends it to a pathology laboratory where it is examined grossly and microscopically in order to make a diagnosis. A knife or scalpel is the instrument usually used.

Where are biopsies most likely to be taken?

In hospitals or in physicians' offices.

What is meant by a needle biopsy?

This is a test whereby a needle is placed into a diseased area and cells or contents are withdrawn and examined by the pathologist.

Is a needle biopsy as accurate as an ordinary biopsy?

Usually not, because the amount of tissue that can be obtained with the needle is so small that it makes interpretation difficult.

What is an incisional biopsy?

It means taking a scalpel and cutting into a diseased area and removing a portion. This fragment is subjected to gross and microscopic examination by the pathologist, who then makes a diagnosis.

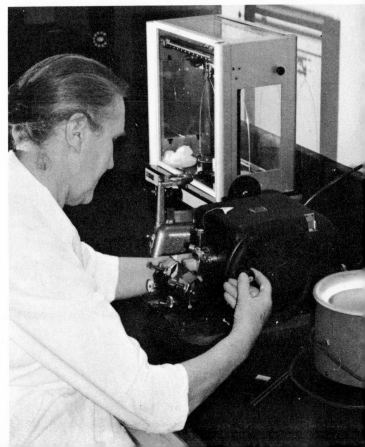

This photograph shows a laboratory technician cutting tissues prior to making a microscopic section for tissue analysis.

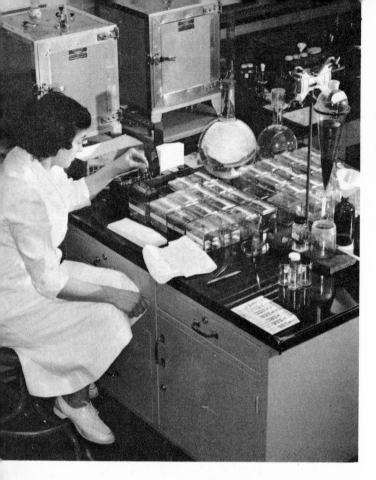

What is meant by an excisional biopsy?

This means removing the entire diseased area, which is then submitted to gross and microscopic examination by the pathologist.

What is meant by a "frozen section"?

This means taking tissue from the patient while the patient is on the operating table and having it immediately submitted to microscopic examination by the pathologist.

Are frozen section examinations infallible?

No. The methods by which the tissues are frozen and subjected to immediate microscopic examination are not as accurate as the usual, more time-consuming methods of preparing tissues for examination in a pathology laboratory.

What is the value of a frozen section examination?

It will tell the surgeon whether a diseased area is malignant or not, thus indicating whether or not a more extensive operation is necessary.

When are frozen sections particularly useful?

In determining whether a mass in the breast is cancerous.

When the pathologist is called into the operating room, will he always be able to know immediately whether or not a tissue is malignant?

No. If there is the slightest doubt in his mind, he will recommend that the more extensive operation be withheld for a day or two until a final report can be obtained on the tissue, after more extensive study under the microscope.

Do pathology laboratories prepare vaccines?

Certain types of vaccines, when obtained from the bacteria of the patient himself, are prepared in pathology laboratories. Commercial vaccines can be bought in drugstores.

What is an autogenous vaccine?

This is a suspension of killed bacteria prepared for the patient from germs which have been freshly isolated from his own body. It is used in an attempt to build up the patient's resistance against these germs.

In what conditions are autogenous vaccines often prepared?

In cases of stubborn recurring infections, such as infections of the urinary tract, and for patients who have recurrent abscesses and boils.

SPUTUM ANALYSIS

Why is sputum analysis carried out?

a. For determining the presence or absence of the germ causing tuberculosis or other lung infections.
b. For analysis in certain cases of asthma.
c. For determining the presence or absence of malignant cells in possible cancer of the lung.

How is the sputum analyzed?

Concentrated smears are made and these are examined carefully under the microscope by the pathologist. Cultures are made to isolate the offending bacteria.

STOOL ANALYSIS

For what conditions is the stool analyzed?

a. For any of the diarrheal diseases, such as dysentery, etc.

b. In cases of sprue or celiac disease.

c. In cases of anemia, if the cause has not been determined through other means.

Bacterial Culture. This is a photograph of an actual laboratory culture showing living colonies of bacteria. This plate proves that the pus taken from an abscess of a patient contains active, live, growing bacteria. By noting the various characteristics of these bacteria and by placing them on a slide and examining them under a microscope, it is possible to determine exactly which bacteria is the cause of the infection.

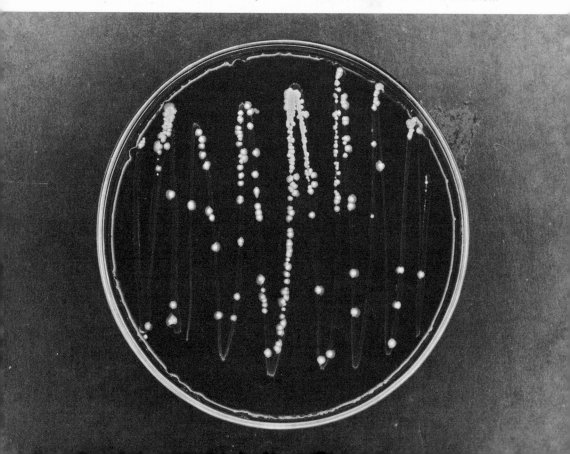

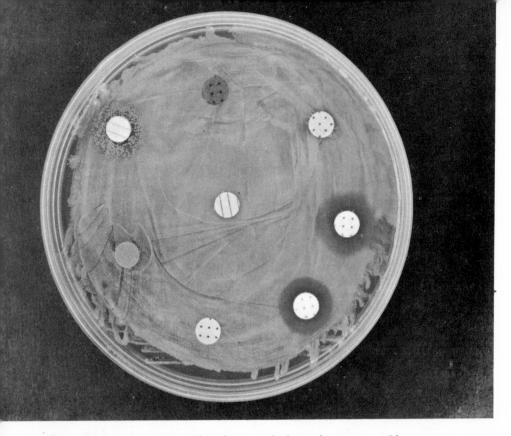

Antibiotic Sensitivity Tests.   This photograph shows the reaction of bacteria to various antibiotic drugs. The gray background in the large circle is bacterial growth; the small spots are bits of cloth soaked with different drugs; the dark rings around the two lower right discs are clear areas showing that those particular antibiotics have prevented bacteria from growing. The bacteria are not sensitive to the other antibiotics.

Is it important for a fresh specimen to be analyzed?

Yes. The specimen has to be brought to the laboratory almost immediately after it has been passed; otherwise the bacteria, parasites, enzymes, etc., in the stool may be lost.

PUS CULTURES

Why are cultures made from pus?

It is very important when pus has been evacuated from the body to determine the particular germ which has produced the infection.

How is this done by the pathology laboratory?

By growing the germs on appropriate culture media.

What is the advantage of finding out the particular germ which has caused an infection?

The treatment rendered will be dictated by the exact nature of the germ which has caused the infection. Different germs vary in their susceptibility to drugs; the appropriate drug must be used to combat a given infecting organism.

LUNG TAPS
(Thoracentesis)

Why is a lung tap performed?

a. To remove fluid which may have accumulated in the chest cavity.
b. To determine whether a germ has caused a pleurisy, and to identify it.
c. To determine the presence or absence of any malignant cells in a case of possible cancer of the lung or in the coverings of the lung.

Are lung taps painful?

There is very little pain. A local injection of novocaine will probably be given before the needle is inserted.

Where are lung taps carried out?

Either in the laboratory, the doctor's office, or the hospital.

ABDOMINAL TAPS
(Paracentesis)

Why are abdominal taps carried out?

a. To remove fluid which may have accumulated in the abdominal cavity.
b. To determine the presence or absence of bacteria which may have caused a peritonitis.
c. To determine the presence or absence of malignant cells.

Is an abdominal tap painful?

The pain is not very great, as some local anesthesia will be given before the needle is inserted into the abdominal cavity.

SPINAL TAPS

What is a spinal tap?

It is a procedure wherein a needle is inserted in the back into the spinal canal and spinal fluid is withdrawn.

Why are spinal taps carried out?

a. To determine the presence or absence of infection within the spinal fluid and brain coverings.
b. To determine the presence or absence of increased pressure within the spinal canal which may be caused by the presence of a tumor of the spinal cord or brain.
c. To instill air or opaque substances prior to examining the spinal cord and brain by x-ray for the presence or absence of tumors or other disease.

Is a spinal tap painful?

No. It causes only slight discomfort, as it is common practice to inject novocaine into the sensitive structures prior to inserting the needle into the spinal canal.

GUINEA PIG INOCULATIONS

What are guinea pig inoculations used for?

Material is taken from a patient's body and is injected into a guinea pig in order to determine the presence or absence of tuberculosis.

How long does it take for a report to be given when a guinea pig inoculation has been carried out?

It takes approximately six weeks.

35

The Lips, Jaws, Mouth, Teeth, and Tongue

THE LIPS

Why do the lips swell so much after even a slight injury?

Because the tissues beneath the skin in this region are elastic and spongy, thus permitting the collection of large amounts of blood.

What is the treatment for swollen lips due to bruises or other injuries?

Apply cold applications and direct pressure as soon as possible after the injury. Most of the swelling will subside within a few days without treatment.

Is it advisable to have a surgeon suture severe lacerations of the lip?

Yes. Cuts about the lips should be stitched expertly, so that an ugly scar will not result.

Are infections about the lips, such as boils, pimples, or carbuncles, dangerous?

Yes, especially those around the nose, cheeks, and upper lip. This is a source of danger, if improperly handled, because the blood vessels in this area of the face drain into veins at the base of the brain. Extension of an infection along this channel may lead to an infection within or surrounding the brain.

What is the most important precaution in the treatment of an infection of the lip?

Never open or squeeze an infected pimple or boil on a lip!

What is the treatment for lip infections?

Small pimples are best left alone. The larger infections are treated by giving the antibiotic drugs and by applying hot, wet compresses to the area. Infections of the lip, especially the upper lip, should be opened only by a surgeon.

Can a syphilitic infection of the lip result from kissing an infected person?

Yes. In former years, chancres of the lip were seen quite often.

Should one avoid kissing a person with a sore on the lip?

Definitely, yes!

Are tumors of the lip common?

Yes. They usually take the form of small, wartlike growths (papillomas), bluish blood vessel tumors (hemangiomas), small freckle-like moles (nevus) of the colored part of the lip, small firm nodules caused by fibrous tissue (fibromas), small retention cysts from one of the glands of the lip, or cancer.

What is the treatment for tumors of the lip?

All of the above-mentioned tumors, except cancer, are benign. They should be removed surgically if they are subject to constant irritation or if they show signs of growth. They are variously treated by surgical excision, by being burned off with an electric needle, by the use of dry ice, or by the application of radium or x-ray therapy. The type of treatment will depend upon the kind of tumor encountered. It is very important that treatment be performed by an expert, so that a minimal scar will result.

Is cancer of the lip common?

Yes. It comprises 2 per cent of all cancer in the body, about 30 per cent of all cancer about the oral cavity.

Who is most likely to be afflicted with cancer of the lip?

Approximately 95 per cent of all cases are in men, and the lower lip is involved in nine out of ten cases.

What is thought to be a major contributing cause of cancer of the lip?

Smoking, particularly of pipes; lip biting; overexposure to the sun; overexposure to wind and adverse weather conditions. Also, any recurrent irritant which comes into contact with the lip is likely to be a predisposing cause for the development of cancer.

What is the appearance of cancer of the lip?

It may look like a wart, a sore which fails to heal, or a cyst.

What is the treatment for cancer of the lip?

Any suspicious chronic sore or lesion of the lip should be removed and submitted for microscopic examination. If a frank cancer has been found, it should be widely excised by a wedge-shaped excision of the sore and surrounding normal tissue.

Is x-ray therapy, radium treatment, or excision with an electric needle ever used instead of surgery?

Yes, but only on rare occasions.

What are the results of surgery for cancer of the lip?

When surgery takes place early, before spread to the glands in the neck, cure is the usual outcome. If spread has already reached the glands in the neck, a more extensive excision is carried out and a radical neck dissection is performed, with removal of all the lymph glands and surrounding tissues.

Is cancer of the lip curable?

Definitely, yes, when discovered in its early stages. The great majority of cancers of the lip can be removed by wide local excision before they have extended to the glands of the neck. Even if the tumor has extended to the glands in the neck, competent radical surgery can produce a cure.

Is the local removal of a cancer of the lip disfiguring?

Not usually. It is surprising how little deformity results from even the removal of 30 to 40 per cent of the lip. Of course, these procedures must be carried out by surgeons who understand the cosmetic aspects of this type of surgery.

Harelip — (label pointing to illustration)

Harelip. This is a rather uncommon birth deformity. Fortunately, plastic surgery can repair this deformity so that it becomes barely visible. It is wise to operate soon after birth, to enable the child to nurse normally.

HARELIP

What is harelip?

It is an open or cleft upper lip with which a child is born.

Does the lower lip ever show a cleft?

Only in very rare instances.

What causes harelip?

Failure of the two sides of the upper lip to fuse during the development of the embryo.

How often does harelip occur?

About once in every thousand births.

Does harelip tend to run in families?

Yes.

What is the treatment for harelip?

Surgical restoration of the lip to normal appearance and function is performed as soon as the infant has shown evidences of gaining weight, and is able to stabilize himself on a feeding formula.

At what age can harelip operations be performed?

Preferably within the first few weeks of life. Because the presence of a harelip in an infant may have a bad psychological effect on other children in the family, it is advisable, if possible, to have the operation performed even before taking the baby home from the hospital.

What is the actual surgical procedure for repair of harelip?

The meticulous and accurate suturing of the separated tissues, layer by layer, so that not only are the external skin surfaces stitched to one another but also the underlying tissues.

What are the results of harelip operations?

They are almost always functionally excellent; cosmetically, they will leave a small thin scar which will tend to fade as the child grows older.

CLEFT PALATE

What is cleft palate?

A malformation of the roof of the mouth of the newborn child which allows open communication between the nose and the mouth. The cleft, or separation, may extend through the hard and soft palate in the complete type, or may involve only the soft palate.

What causes cleft palate?

It is a malformation during the growth of the embryo which is

Cleft Palate. This deformity is sometimes associated with hare-lip. Cleft palate is somewhat more difficult to cure surgically, but most children, by the time they are two to three years of age, can be successfully treated by surgery.

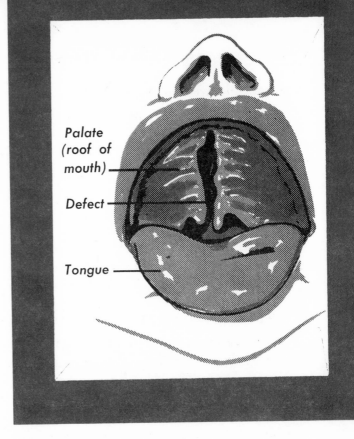

Palate (roof of mouth)

Defect

Tongue

thought to take place somewhere between the sixth and twelfth week of development.

Does cleft palate tend to run in families?

Yes, but present-day investigators feel that some disease such as German measles, which the mother may develop during early pregnancy, is also a factor in the development of this and other deformities.

How often does cleft palate occur?

Possibly once in every thousand births.

Does cleft palate interfere with normal feeding?

Yes. Food and liquids are pushed through the defect up into the nose during the course of swallowing.

Will a cleft palate interfere with speaking?

Yes. Normal sounds of speech cannot be developed, as there is a loss of the resonating factor of the closed palate.

What is the treatment for cleft palate?

Surgical correction to overcome the defective fusion of the palate and to develop normal function for speech and eating purposes. The operative procedures are often performed in successive stages for the more extended conditions and require very expert and special surgery.

At what age should operations for cleft palate be performed?

In an occasional case, it can be done as early as the first few months of life; other children should be operated on anywhere between the ages of one and a half and three years, or later in some cases.

Who should perform operations for cleft palate?

It is a team function and will often demand the cooperation of the oral surgeon, the plastic surgeon, and the dental surgeon.

Is follow-up care essential after operations for cleft palate?

Yes. Psychologists and speech instructors are often necessary to teach the child the normal use of his voice after operations of this type.

Are operations for cleft palate successful?

Yes, but failures of one particular operation are encountered often. It must be remembered that several operations may be necessary over a period of years in order to bring about an eventual cure.

THE JAWS

What are the common conditions affecting the jaws?

a. Infection. Infections of the bones of the jaw are usually secondary to infected teeth. Such infections (osteomyelitis) are seen much less often since the advent of the antibiotic drugs.
b. Fractures of the jaws.
c. Cysts or tumors of the jaws.

What is the treatment for an infection of the jaws?

Infection of the bones of the jaw, as mentioned above, occurs from abscessed teeth or, in rare instances, from an infected sinus. The treatment may involve the expert use of the antibiotic drugs and, in occasional cases, surgical drainage and removal of infected bone.

Are bone infections of the jaws serious?

Yes, but with newer methods, eventual recovery over a period of time will result.

Are fractures of the jaw common?

Yes, particularly with the increasing number of auto accidents taking place today.

What are the symptoms of a fractured jaw?

Pain, swelling, tenderness, difficulty in chewing, loose or missing teeth, and bleeding from the mouth. When the fragments of the fracture are displaced, the patient may find himself unable to close his mouth properly. In fractures of the upper jaw, air may become trapped under the skin, and the front of the face may become swollen, particularly under the eyes.

When one notes a fracture of the jaw, is there often an accompanying fracture of the skull?

Yes. The injury which has produced the jaw fracture often has also produced damage to the bones of the skull.

Where do jaw fractures usually take place?

In the lower jaw, they occur most commonly in the center at the level of the premolar teeth. The upper jaw usually breaks transversely, with loosening of the teeth, and also involves the maxillary sinus.

Who should treat fractured jaws?

Oral surgeons, often in conjunction with nose and throat surgeons or plastic surgeons.

What is the treatment for fractured jaw?

In the uncomplicated case, first-aid treatment aims to immobilize the

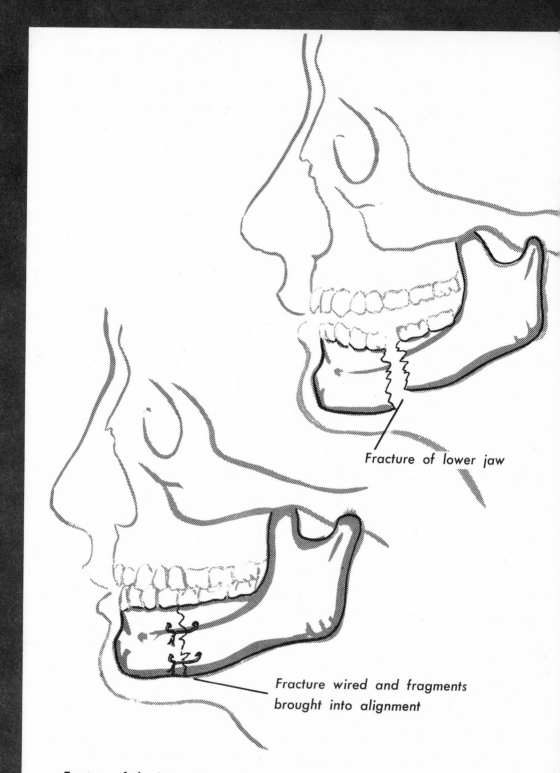

Fracture of lower jaw

Fracture wired and fragments brought into alignment

Fracture of the Lower Jaw. The fracture has been wired and the fragments have been brought into alignment. Most of these conditions are treated by an oral surgeon or by one who specializes in conditions about the face. Orthopedists do not usually treat fractured jaws.

jaw, either with handkerchief or bandage. Definitive treatment aims at immobilizing the jaws by wiring the teeth together after setting the deformity. The upper teeth are often wired to the lower teeth in order to keep the jaws splinted or closed.

Is it ever necessary to operate for fracture of the jaw?

Yes. In the more complicated case, particularly in the compound fracture, it is often necessary to perform an operation within the mouth and to nail or pin the fragments together. Where bone has been lost, a bone graft may be taken or a metal plate may be used to make up for lost fragments.

How does a patient eat when the jaws are wired together?

It is often necessary to limit the patient to a completely liquid diet so long as the jaws are wired together.

How long do fractures of the jaw take to heal?

Anywhere from four to six weeks.

Is hospitalization necessary for fractured jaw?

The simple cases can be handled in the office of the oral surgeon, but severe cases must be hospitalized and anesthesia given if they require operative intervention.

Are cysts of the jaws common?

Yes. Malformation of the teeth, with failure of the tooth to emerge beyond the jaw margins, often leads to the formation of cysts. These are called dentigerous cysts.

What is the treatment for cysts of the jaw?

The oral surgeon must open the bone overlying the cyst and remove the tooth. The cyst will then fill in with bone.

Are malignant tumors of the jaw common?

No. When they are encountered they require wide removal of the jaw bones. These procedures must be carried out by surgeons who specialize in this type of work (maxillofacial surgeons).

THE MOUTH

What causes bad breath?

The condition may be transitory and may develop after eating certain foods, taking certain medications, or after excessive smoking or drinking of alcoholic beverages. Under these circumstances, all one has to do is remove the inciting cause. Local disease within the mouth, such as infected or poorly cared for teeth—or infected gums—may also cause bad breath. Generalized disease such as gastro-intestinal illness, or diseases of the lungs or liver or kidneys, may also result in bad breath.

What is the treatment for bad breath?

Since there are innumerable possible causes, it requires a thorough investigation to eliminate the condition. Any local disease within the mouth should be corrected, and proper hygiene of the teeth should be instituted. A general examination by a physician is warranted in such cases in order to rule out general disease.

What can be done locally to cut down on bad breath?

Oral hygiene should be maintained. Consult your dentist for treatment of any possible infected teeth or gums. The usual mouthwashes and other measures are usually of a temporary nature in helping to eliminate bad breath.

What is pyorrhea?

An infection along the upper margin of the gums, involving the margin of the teeth with the gums.

What causes pyorrhea?

A bacterial infection of the mouth, frequently with a streptococcus. Local causes permitting infection to take place usually involve improper bite, poor dental hygiene, tartar formation, improper and infrequent brushing of the teeth, irritation by smoking, or the excessive use of alcohol. Certain deficiency diseases, such as the vitamin-deficiency diseases, may also be accompanied by pyorrhea.

What are the signs of pyorrhea?

Redness and sponginess, with bleeding from the gums. Also, there may be frank yellow pus formation at the base of the teeth.

What is the treatment for pyorrhea?

Treatment by a competent dentist is necessary in order to remove tartar and to correct any other dental defects. He will undoubtedly prescribe local medications which will help in obliterating the infection.

Is pyorrhea curable?

Yes, but treatment is often prolonged and requires rehabilitation of the mouth cavity.

What is trench mouth?

Trench mouth, or Vincent's angina, is a frequently encountered specific infection and inflammation of the lining of the mouth caused by a specific germ.

How does one get trench mouth?

It is usually spread by direct contact with an infected person or by using articles, such as eating utensils, used by a contaminated person.

Can trench mouth be transmitted by kissing?

Yes.

Does trench mouth ever affect the tonsils and the throat as well as the mouth?

Yes.

What are the symptoms of trench mouth?

If it is localized, the patient may complain of a bad taste in the mouth, and those surrounding him may note a bad odor to his breath. There may be small, painful ulcerations on the tongue or inner aspect of the lips or gums which may produce some bleeding.

Can trench mouth cause swollen glands in the neck?

Yes, and it may also cause fever.

What is the treatment for trench mouth?

a. Avoid contact with others, as this is a highly contagious disease.

b. Antibiotics, particularly the proper usage of penicillin.

c. Local application of the proper medications to the ulcerations, and the local use of a mouthwash.

LEUKOPLAKIA

Is there any other name for leukoplakia?

Yes. It is frequently called smoker's tongue, smoker's patches, etc.

What is leukoplakia?

The word means white plate. It is manifested as a disease appearing on the mucous membranes or lining of the oral cavity and presents itself as whitish or whitish-blue thickenings on the inner aspects of the cheeks, palate, gums, tongue, wall of the pharynx, and sometimes the larynx. These patches are sometimes elevated, roughened, or bark-like.

What causes leukoplakia?

The exact cause is not known, but its high incidence among smokers suggests that local irritation in the mouth from smoking is a strong contributory factor. Also, roughened tooth edges, poorly fitting dentures, etc., are thought to predispose to leukoplakia.

Who is most likely to be afflicted with leukoplakia?

It is seen more often in men than in women—particularly between the ages of twenty and sixty. However, since smoking has become so fashionable among women, the incidence of the condition is on the rise in that sex.

What are the symptoms of leukoplakia?

Often, there are none at all, and the condition may be noticed accidentally by the patient himself or by the dentist or physician. Occasionally, there is burning and tingling and cracking in a leukoplakic plaque.

What is the significance of leukoplakia?

It is of great significance because it is supposedly a forerunner of cancer. This is one of the definite instances in medicine where a non-cancerous condition (such as leukoplakia) can lead to malignant degeneration.

What is the treatment for leukoplakia?

a. Stop smoking.
b. Remove all possible sources of local irritation, such as poorly fitting dentures or roughened skin edges.
c. Removal of the leukoplakic patch either by an electric needle or by surgical excision of the area.

Is hospitalization necessary for removal of areas of leukoplakia?

The great majority of these cases can be treated adequately in the surgeon's office by treatment with an electric needle. However, when patches must be removed from the throat or from the larynx, hospitalization is advised.

Can successful treatment of leukoplakia avoid the development of cancer?

Yes. People with leukoplakia should be kept under constant supervision so that the progress of the disease can be noted.

THE TEETH

What causes cavities of the teeth?

The specific cause is not actually known, but it is thought that a chemical decalcification is stimulated by the action of certain acid-producing bacteria or germs which grow in the mouth. Improper diet and improper hygiene also predispose to cavity formation. Also, irritation of the teeth by poor bite or by poorly fitting dentures are thought to cause cavities.

What is the best way to prevent cavities of the teeth?

Dental examination at regular intervals. Also, the maintenance of proper dental hygiene and attention to one's general health.

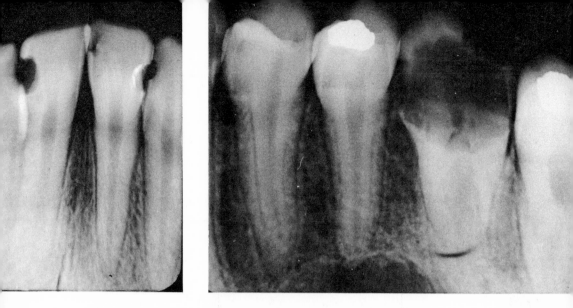

Left: X-rays Showing Cavities in the Teeth. These are relatively small cavities and these teeth can be saved by having them drilled and filled.

Right: Tooth Decay. These x-rays show a decayed tooth which will probably have to be removed and other teeth with cavities that have already been filled. All adults should have their teeth examined once a year, as cavities can form within a period of a few months.

Can the presence of diseased teeth affect the general health of a patient?

Yes. The teeth are part of the human body and infection or disease within the teeth can spread to other parts of the body.

How can one tell if he has an abscessed tooth?

Abscessed teeth are almost always accompanied by a local reaction involving swelling, pain, and redness in the area. A chronic abscess, however, may not be readily discernible by the patient.

What is the treatment for an abscessed tooth?

See your dentist. He will usually prescribe antibiotics and, in most instances, will have to remove the infected tooth.

Can bacteria affecting the teeth spread to other parts of the body?

Yes. This is particularly important to avoid in people who have disease of the heart. It is known that people with valvular disease of the heart may develop an infection on those diseased valves from infected teeth.

THE TONGUE

What is glossitis?

It is an inflammation of the tongue.

Is the tongue often involved in an infection or inflammation or true abscess formation?

No. The tongue is peculiarly immune to the formation of abscesses. This may possibly be attributed to its very rich blood supply.

What is the treatment for inflammations of the tongue?

Since glossitis is usually a sign or a symptom of disease elsewhere, the treatment will depend upon the causative factor. Whenever a local irritant is causing a change in the tongue, this must be eliminated.

Is the tongue subject to many changes in its appearance?

Yes. The tongue has been used for generations by physicians to make various diagnoses of general diseases. The tongue may be swollen or reddened or whitish or smoother than normal, and may change its appearance from day to day.

What local factors often produce changes in the appearance of the tongue?

Tobacco, alcohol, highly spiced foods, or excessively hot foods may cause a tongue to look red and irritated. The edge of the tongue may be irritated by rough, sharp edges of teeth or improperly fitted dentures. Also, the tongue may be affected by infections within the mouth, such as trench mouth, syphilis, etc. Vitamin deficiencies, too, may alter the appearance of the tongue.

What general diseases of the body are most frequently reflected in changes of the appearance of the tongue?

Deficiency diseases, such as certain types of anemia (pernicious anemia). Also, generalized skin conditions will give a characteristic appearance to the tongue.

What condition of the body is most closely reflected in the appearance of the tongue?

The state of hydration or dehydration. The tongue appears dry and coated whenever the patient lacks the proper amount of fluids within his body.

Is the tongue often the site of tumor formation?

Yes.

What are the common tumors of the tongue?

a. Leukoplakia. This is really not a true tumor but is a forerunner of tumor formation.

b. Blood vessel tumors (hemangioma).

c. Wart-like tumors (papillomas).

d. Gland cell tumors (adenomas).

e. Connective tissue tumors (fibromas).

f. Cysts of the tongue occasionally caused by failure of the thyroid gland to develop fully (thyroglossal cysts).

g. Cancer of the tongue.

Is cancer of the tongue a common condition?

Yes. It comprises about one out of five of all cancers within the oral cavity.

Where is cancer of the tongue usually seen?

Along the tongue margins or at the edge of the tongue.

Does cancer of the tongue affect men more than women?

Yes—by a ratio of eight to one.

At what age is cancer of the tongue most frequently encountered?

Between forty and sixty years of age.

What causes cancer of the tongue?

It is not definitely known, but it is thought that the common factor of chronic recurrent irritation may be a predisposing factor. It must be strongly emphasized that the greatest incidence of cancer of the tongue is seen among pipe smokers. The second most common predisposing cause of cancer of the tongue appears to be sharp edges of the teeth, poorly fitting dentures, and poor hygiene of the mouth.

How is the diagnosis of cancer of the tongue made?

It has a characteristic appearance which soon makes itself evident to the examining physician. The positive diagnosis is made by removing a small piece of the tissue and submitting it to microscopic examination.

What is the treatment for tumors of the tongue?

Most benign tumors can be removed surgically or can be treated with surgery plus x-ray or radium applications. All benign tumors of the tongue are curable. Early cancers of the tongue can be cured by wide local excision.

Is it ever necessary to remove the entire tongue for cancer?

Usually, a portion of the tongue is left behind when a cancer is found. However, if the cancer has already spread to the glands in the neck, a wide radical excision of the tongue and the glands in the neck may produce a cure.

Is surgery always the treatment of choice for cancer of the tongue?

No. There are certain types of cancer, particularly those which occur in the posterior portions of the tongue, which are better treated with radium or x-ray.

What are the chances of cure for cancer of the tongue?

More than half of those cases seen in their early stages can be permanently cured. However, all too often treatment is started late and it is sad to report that cancer of the tongue is responsible for more deaths than any other tumor arising in the head and neck.

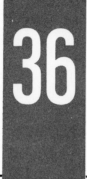 *The Liver*

What is the liver, and where is it located?

The liver is a very large glandular organ of reddish-brown color located in the upper abdominal cavity beneath the diaphragm and ribs. It stretches across the upper abdomen for approximately eight inches, and extends irregularly in shape for six or seven inches in a vertical direction from front to back. It is divided into two lobes, a right and left, the right lobe being about three times the size of the left lobe.

What are the functions of the liver?

The liver is the most important structure in the body in the regulation of chemical reactions. It is not possible to enumerate all of its functions, but the main ones are:

a. The production and storage of proteins, the regulation and control of the many by-products of protein metabolism.

b. The storage of sugar and the regulation of the amount of sugar circulating in the blood.

c. The neutralization of toxic and harmful substances in the body.

d. The utilization and storage of fats.

e. The manufacture of substances important to blood coagulation.

f. The manufacture of bile and bile salts which are secreted through the ducts into the intestines and which aid in digestion.

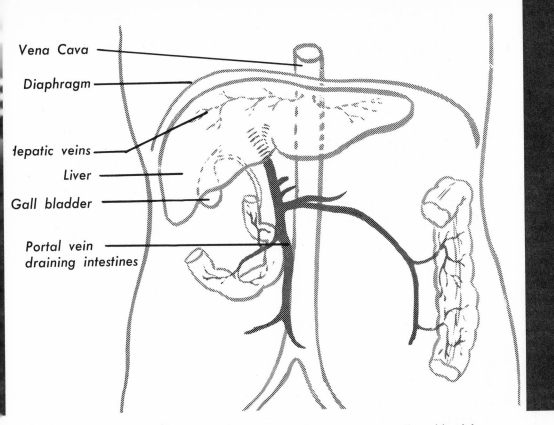

Anatomy of the Liver and the Portal System. The portal vein collects blood from the intestinal tract and transports it to the liver. Through this portal system, food elements which have been absorbed from the intestines are brought to the liver, where their chemical components are extracted.

g. The manufacture and storage of substances important to the production of red blood cells and other components of the blood.

Can a patient survive without a liver?

No. It is essential to life.

What are the usual causes of impairment of liver function?

a. Infection of the liver.

b. Parasite infestation of the liver.

c. Cancerous invasion.

d. Liver poisoning, from the ingestion of poisons or certain medications which may adversely affect the liver.

e. Prolonged obstruction of the bile ducts with obstruction to the outflow of bile.

f. Severe malnutrition.

g. Disturbance in the blood supply to the liver.

h. Replacement of its vital structure by abnormally produced substances, such as amyloid.

i. Upset in liver chemistry.

j. Cirrhosis of the liver (replacement of liver substance by fibrous tissue).

Are diseases of the liver very common?

Yes, but they are not very obvious because the liver has an extraordinary ability to fight off disease and to function satisfactorily despite disease.

Can the liver continue to function satisfactorily when a large portion of its substance is involved in a disease process?

Yes.

Is liver disease easy to diagnose?

No, because serious and progressive liver disease may exist for many years without giving any apparent signs or symptoms to the patient. This is because the liver has a great functional reserve.

How does one go about discovering if there is liver disease?

By careful noting of the patient's history, careful physical examination, and by a variety of laboratory tests performed on the blood, stool, and urine.

What is meant by the terms "biliousness," "torpid liver," and "liverish"?

These are terms used by lay people who believe they may have disease of their liver. More usually, the symptoms are not related to liver upset but are associated with indigestion, dietary indiscretions, emotional disturbance, or perhaps other diseases of the gall bladder or intestinal tract.

What is jaundice?

Jaundice is a generalized yellowish discoloration of the skin and the white of the eyeball due to an abnormally high concentration of bile pigments in the blood.

Does jaundice always indicate liver disease?

No. It may be due to excessive destruction of red blood cells by disease involving the blood itself. Or it may be due to damming back of the bile into the bloodstream because of disease of the gall bladder, bile ducts, pancreas, or other organs adjacent to the liver. This latter type of jaundice is called "obstructive jaundice."

What is acute yellow atrophy of the liver?

This term signifies rapid and progressive destruction of the liver as a result of infection or chemical poisoning. The condition is accompanied by a severe degree of jaundice and by a shrinking or death of many of the liver cells. Usually, this condition is rapidly fatal.

Can heart disease affect the liver?

Yes. With a poorly functioning or failing heart, the liver may become enlarged and engorged with stagnated blood. If this situation persists over a prolonged period of time, permanent liver injury may result.

Do gallstones ever cause liver damage?

Yes, by obstructing the bile ducts and the flow of bile into the intestines, the bile is dammed back into the liver substance. This may result in grave damage to liver function and to the liver cells themselves. Such a condition, if persistent, may cause biliary cirrhosis.

Is the liver ever afflicted with bacterial infection?

Yes. Bacteria may set up infection within the liver, either generalized or in the form of an abscess or abscesses. This may occur as a complication of other diseases, such as pneumonia, typhoid fever, appendicitis, etc. These complications are relatively rare today because of the effective treatment of the primary disease with antibiotic drugs.

Can infectious mononucleosis (glandular fever) cause liver disease?

Yes. The patient may develop the same clinical picture as seen in infectious hepatitis. The condition usually clears up completely and leaves no residual liver damage.

Do parasites ever infest the liver?

Yes. A wide variety of parasites may find their way to the liver, either through having been eaten in contaminated foods or water, or by penetrating the skin of a person bathing in infested waters. This occurs much more frequently in tropical climates outside of the United States—in the Orient, Africa, the Philippine Islands, etc.

CIRRHOSIS

What is cirrhosis of the liver?

It is a general term meant to signify chronic generalized destruction and scarring of liver tissue, with impairment of liver function to a slight or greater degree.

What causes cirrhosis of the liver?

Any disease process which involves the liver may eventually lead to cirrhosis, that is, destruction of liver cells and replacement by scar tissue.

Can drinking alcohol over a prolonged period of time produce cirrhosis?

Yes. The association between people who drink alcoholic beverages excessively and the occurrence of cirrhosis is well known. It is thought that the liver damage results from the combined effect of the toxic action of the alcohol upon the liver and the poor nutritional intake usually associated with those who drink excessively.

Will drinking in moderation cause cirrhosis of the liver?

No, but of course this involves a definition of the term "moderate drinking." An occasional highball or drink before dinner is not likely to cause liver damage, especially when the diet and food intake is adequate. However, the tolerance to the toxic effects of alcohol varies widely from one individual to another.

What are the symptoms of cirrhosis?

These vary with the degree of liver destruction and liver reserve. Many cases go undetected and without symptoms for years. As liver function deteriorates, it may be accompanied by loss of appetite, nausea, vomiting, and weight loss. There may be abdominal discomfort, fullness in the upper abdomen, and indigestion. When the disease progresses, there may be a listlessness and weakness, with loss of energy. When extensive liver destruction has taken place, the legs and abdomen may become swollen with fluid (dropsy), jaundice may come on, and the patient's mental state may become confused and disoriented. The final outcome may be coma and death.

Is cirrhosis always fatal?

No. If it is detected at an early stage, and if proper treatment is carried out, a patient with cirrhosis may live his normal span of years.

How is cirrhosis of the liver diagnosed?

By studying the patient's history and by physical examination, as well as by certain laboratory tests performed upon the blood, urine, and stool.

Is the liver always enlarged in cirrhosis?

No. During the later stages it may become shrunken and smaller than normal.

Is the spleen often enlarged in cirrhosis of the liver?

Yes.

How is cirrhosis of the liver treated?

First, it is important to remove any toxic influences, such as infection, obstruction to the outflow of bile, or liver poisons that the patient may be taking. Next, there must be a satisfactory dietary intake, with the proper amounts of minerals and vitamins.

Is cirrhosis ever complicated by hemorrhage?

Yes. Varicosed veins within the esophagus will frequently bleed in cases of advanced cirrhosis. This is caused by these veins becoming swollen because they carry blood which ordinarily would have gone through the liver had it not been involved in cirrhosis.

FATTY LIVER

What is a fatty liver?

A fatty liver is one which has many times the normal component of fat.

What is the cause of fatty liver?

It is caused by malnutrition, alcoholism, marked anemia, diabetes, or chemical poisoning.

What are the symptoms of fatty liver?

Usually there are none, except for enlargement of the liver. However, if the underlying cause is not removed, severe and progressive damage to the liver may occur.

What is the treatment of fatty liver?

Elimination of the basic cause, then giving a well-balanced diet, with proper vitamin and mineral supplements.

CANCER OF THE LIVER

Is the liver ever involved in cancer?

Yes. There may be a primary cancer, in which the cells of the liver themselves originate the cancer; or there may be metastatic involvement of the liver, in which the cancer cells have originated elsewhere in the body.

What causes primary cancer of the liver?

The cause is not really known, but it has been found that a considerable number of cases develop in those livers which have been previously cirrhotic. In addition, certain chemical toxins and parasitic infestations have been incriminated in a small percentage of these cases.

Is it common for the liver to be involved in cancer which has originated elsewhere?

Yes. The liver is the organ most commonly involved by cancer which has spread from another organ, such as the stomach, pancreas, gall bladder, breast, kidney, or intestines.

What are the symptoms of cancer of the liver?

These vary widely, depending upon the extent and nature of the involvement as well as upon how the other organs of the body are involved. Usually, there is loss of weight, weakness, loss of appetite, and nodular enlargement of the liver. Eventually, all the symptoms of typical severe liver damage ensue—such as jaundice, hemorrhage, swelling of the legs, with eventual coma and death.

Can cancer of the liver ever be treated effectively by surgery?

Yes, in an occasional case in which there is involvement of but one lobe (segment) of the organ. New techniques have been developed whereby one half of the liver can be removed surgically.

INFECTIOUS HEPATITIS

What is infectious hepatitis?

This is a common type of infection of the liver which may occur in epidemics and is caused by a virus infection.

Are there any other names for infectious hepatitis?

It is also called epidemic hepatitis, catarrhal jaundice, or hepatitis A.

Who is most likely to develop infectious hepatitis?

Young people seem to be most prone to this condition.

793

Is infectious hepatitis very common?

Yes, and it has been increasing greatly in incidence within the past few years.

What are thought to be some of the causes of an epidemic of infectious hepatitis?

Poor sanitation, contaminated food or water, crowding, and malnutrition.

What are the symptoms of infectious hepatitis?

Over a period of a few days, the patient begins to feel ill, loses energy, loses appetite, feels nauseated, and develops a slight fever. There then ensues tenderness and enlargement of the liver, some pain in the right upper portion of the abdomen, and eventually— about the fifth or sixth day—onset of jaundice. There may also be a gastro-intestinal upset, with vomiting and diarrhea.

Does jaundice always accompany infectious hepatitis?

No. In a small percentage of cases actual jaundice does not occur.

How is a diagnosis of infectious hepatitis made?

By noting the history and symptoms; by finding a tender, enlarged liver; by noting the presence of jaundice; and by characteristic findings on laboratory tests of blood, stool, and urine.

Can infectious hepatitis be distinguished from other liver diseases by special laboratory tests?

Yes.

How long is one usually ill with infectious hepatitis?

Anywhere from six to twelve weeks.

Is it necessary for the patient with infectious hepatitis to stay in bed?

Definitely, yes. The liver is a large organ, and when it is inflamed and infected it must have rest. This can be obtained only in bed.

Does a relapse of infectious hepatitis ever take place?

Yes, in about one out of ten patients, if the patient gets out of bed too soon or resumes activity before he has fully recovered.

Are there any other causes for a relapse of infectious hepatitis?

Yes; poor diet or the drinking of alcoholic beverages.

Are there any specific drugs or antibiotics which are of value in treating infectious hepatitis?

No. Rest and an adequate well-balanced diet are the best forms of treatment.

What are the chances for recovery from infectious hepatitis?

The chances are excellent, although a small percentage of patients, those who do not take care of themselves properly or who have other illnesses, may die. Fortunately, this is a very small percentage of those who get the disease.

Is infectious hepatitis classified as a contagious disease?

Yes. It can be spread by close contact with a patient who is ill with hepatitis. However, the degree of contagion is relatively mild.

Does infectious hepatitis usually cause permanent liver damage?

No. In the vast majority of cases, complete recovery of liver function takes place.

Is there a tendency toward getting another attack of hepatitis once a patient has fully recovered?

No.

Can infectious hepatitis ever become a chronic disease?

Yes. If it is not properly taken care of, permanent liver damage may result.

Can infectious hepatitis be prevented if one has been exposed to a patient who has the disease?

Yes. Gamma globulin injection has been found to be effective in preventing the disease if given early enough after exposure. This protection lasts only four to six weeks. After this passage of time, a repeat exposure may cause the disease unless another injection of gamma globulin is given.

Does gamma globulin have any value in the actual treatment of infectious hepatitis?

No.

SERUM HEPATITIS
(*Homologous Serum Jaundice*)

What is serum hepatitis?

An infection of the liver caused by a virus presumably different from the germ causing infectious hepatitis.

How does one contract serum hepatitis (homologous serum jaundice)?

It is transmitted through receiving a transfusion of blood or plasma, or by contamination from an infected hypodermic needle or syringe.

Is serum hepatitis caused by transfusion of the wrong type of blood?

No.

How long after receiving a blood transfusion or an injection can one contract serum hepatitis?

It takes anywhere from two to six months to develop the disease after one has been inoculated with the virus.

What are the symptoms and course of serum hepatitis (homologous serum jaundice)?

Practically the same symptoms and course as that of infectious hepatitis.

Is serum hepatitis preventable?

Only to a limited extent, by the proper selection of blood donors, proper technique in storing and handling blood and plasma, and by proper sterilization of needles and syringes. However, it must be stated emphatically that even after the above precautions are taken, it is not possible to eliminate entirely the risk of contracting serum hepatitis.

TOXIC HEPATITIS

What is toxic hepatitis?

It is a term used for liver injury caused by taking chemical poisons or drugs which adversely affect the liver.

How does one contract toxic hepatitis?

It may develop rapidly after the inhalation or eating of significant amounts of chemical poisons or drugs, or it may develop gradually over a period of years as a result of prolonged consummation or inhalation of small amounts of these same toxic substances. There is a great individual variation in the susceptibility to such agents.

Is toxic hepatitis curable?

It depends upon the extent to which the poison has already damaged the liver. If the damage has been mild and reversible, recovery will take place.

SURGERY OF THE LIVER

For what conditions is the liver operated upon?

a. Injuries, such as gunshot wounds, stab wounds, or rupture of the liver due to an accident.
b. Abscesses of the liver, as a complication usually of some other disease within the abdominal cavity or elsewhere in the body.
c. Cysts of the liver, most common of which is the echinoccocus cyst, which is caused by a parasite which infests dogs. Constant contact with a dog can transmit this infection to man.
d. Benign tumors, such as hemangiomas (blood cysts) or lymph tumors such as lymphangiomas.
e. Cancer of the liver, in the occasional instance where only one lobe (segment) is involved and can be removed surgically.
f. Cirrhosis of the liver.

How can one diagnose an injury to the liver?

    a. There will be signs of shock and internal hemorrhage.

    b. There is a history of an external injury.

    c. There may be swelling and tenderness in the right upper portion of the abdomen.

Is it always necessary to operate for an injury to the liver?

No. If the patient does not go into shock and if there is evidence that little bleeding has taken place, it is possible to withhold surgery and await developments.

Is rupture of the liver a serious injury?

Yes. However, many of these patients can be saved by prompt surgery.

Is it necessary to operate on all liver abscesses?

No, because the antibiotic drugs will frequently permit the patient to get well without surgery. However, if there is a large collection of pus within the liver, it must be removed by surgical drainage.

Does recovery usually take place after drainage of a liver abscess?

Yes.

Is it possible to successfully remove benign tumors and cysts of the liver?

Great advances in surgical technique have been made, so that tumors can now be removed from the liver satisfactorily. There are cases on record in which an entire lobe of the liver has been successfully removed.

Is it possible to help a liver surgically if it is extensively involved in a cancer process?

No. Only those in which there are isolated masses can be helped.

What is done surgically to help people with cirrhosis of the liver?

Many of these patients can now be helped largely through surgery. Because cirrhosis prevents much of the blood from coursing through

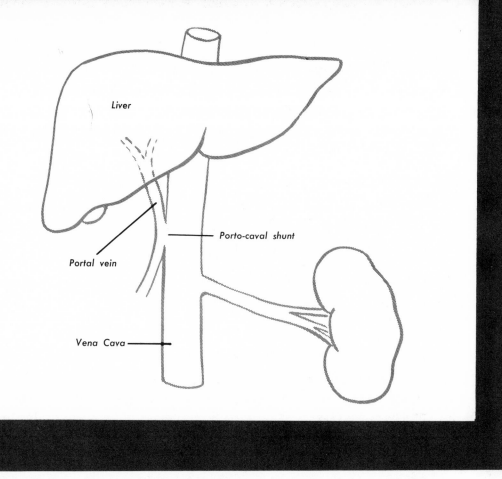

Liver

Portal vein

Porto-caval shunt

Vena Cava

Portocaval Shunt Operation. This diagram shows the joining of the portal vein to the vena cava, thus diverting blood which would ordinarily flow through the liver into the general circulation. This procedure is sometimes necessary for people who have advanced cirrhosis of the liver with obstruction of blood flow.

the liver, operations have been devised which shunt the blood around the liver and thus aid circulation. The two most common operations of this type are:

a. Portocaval shunt, in which the portal vein is stitched to the vena cava. This permits much of the blood to pass directly into the general circulation instead of being held up by a cirrhotic liver.

b. A splenorenal shunt, in which the vein from the spleen is stitched to the left kidney vein. This also allows much of the blood which would ordinarily have gone to the liver to be shunted directly into the general circulation.

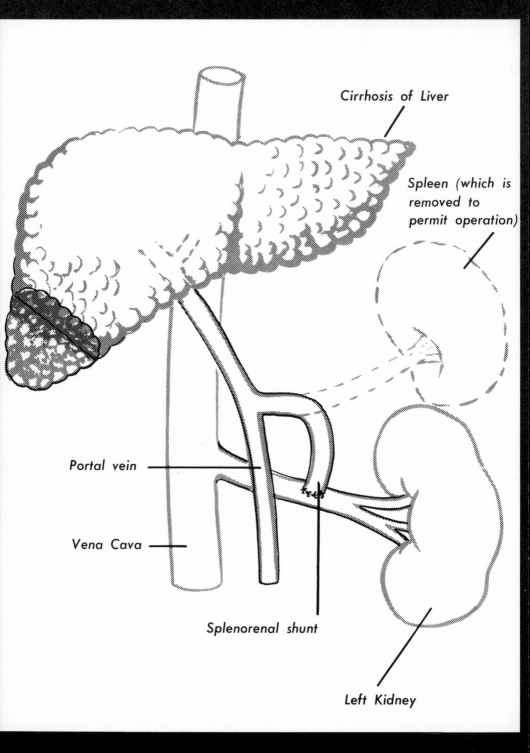

Cirrhosis of Liver

Spleen (which is removed to permit operation)

Portal vein

Vena Cava

Splenorenal shunt

Left Kidney

Splenorenal Shunt Operation. This diagram shows an operation which joins the main vein of the spleen to the renal (kidney) vein, thus shunting blood away from the liver and into the general circulation. This procedure accomplishes the same purpose as the portocaval shunt.

Are operations for cirrhosis of the liver serious?

Yes, but many excellent results have been obtained through these procedures.

What are the chances for improving cirrhosis through these operations?

More than half of these patients are benefited by the shunt operations.

Is it necessary to protect the liver before operating upon diseases of the gall bladder or bile ducts?

Yes. It is important to see that the liver has an adequate supply of sugar to protect it while these structures are being operated upon.

Can one live a normal life after removal of part of the liver?

Yes. Only about one-fifth of the liver substance is necessary to maintain normal function.

Are there accurate tests to determine how badly liver function is impaired?

Yes. There are many blood, urine, and stool tests which will give an accurate picture of what is going on within the liver.

37 *The Lungs*

What is the structure of the lungs?

The lungs are the organs of breathing which are located in the chest cavity. The right lung consists of three sections called lobes, while the left lung has but two lobes. The lungs are composed of spongy tissue surrounding treelike branches of the bronchial tubes. The lung tissue itself consists of innumerable air sacs surrounded by elastic tissue which permits the structure to expand and contract.

What is the function of the lungs?

The lungs take out oxygen from the air that is inhaled, and give up carbon dioxide which has been brought to the lungs by the blood-stream. The carbon dioxide and a certain amount of water in the form of vapor are expelled when one exhales.

Is there such a thing as someone having weak lungs?

No. This expression usually means that the person has some form of lung disease, such as bronchitis or tuberculosis.

Is the tendency toward lung trouble inherited?

No. Lung trouble (usually tuberculosis) occurs in families because of spread from one member to another rather than by inheritance. The parent or grandparent who is not aware that he or she has tuberculosis can spread it to a child or grandchild.

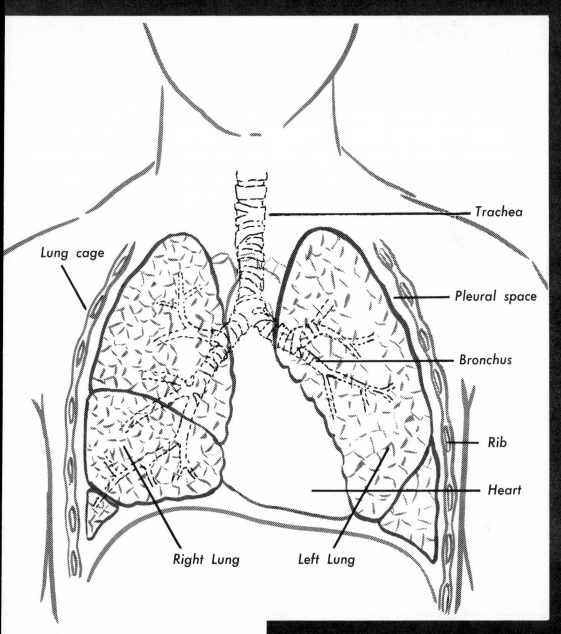

Trachea

Lung cage

Pleural space

Bronchus

Rib

Heart

Right Lung

Left Lung

The Lungs, Chest Cavity, Bronchiectasis. This diagram shows the anatomy of the lungs with its bronchial tubes and air sacs. The insert shows a chronic condition, bronchiectasis, in which the air sacs and small bronchioles are enlarged and irregularly shaped. This disease is serious, as mucous secretions tend to stagnate in the air sacs, and this leads to chronic lung infection. Bronchiectasis can often be cured by removing the diseased portions of lung.

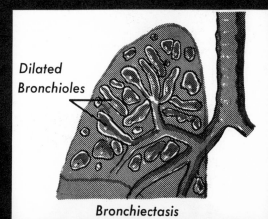

Dilated Bronchioles

Bronchiectasis

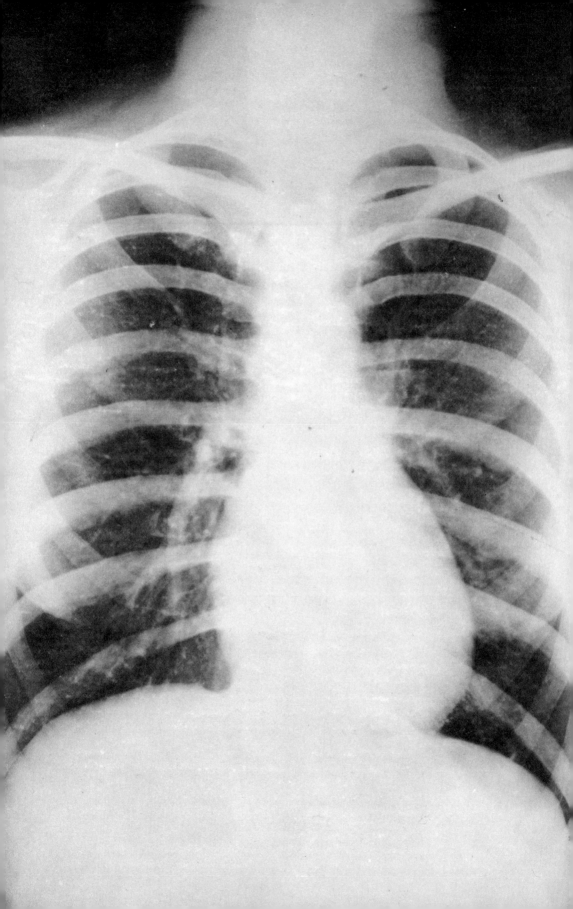

Is it healthier to live in the country where the air is pure, than in the city where the air tends to be impure?

In general, yes. Irritating dusts and fumes are more prevalent in the cities and tend to produce respiratory difficulty in the nose, throat, and in the bronchial tubes.

What conditions can be caused by breathing impure air?

The impurities in the air, such as smoke, fumes, smog, etc., cause irritation of the lining membranes and lower the resistance of these tissues to infection and possibly to tumor formation.

How often should one have his lungs examined?

About once a year. Healthy adults should have chest x-rays about every year or two unless there is some reason for more frequent x-rays.

Can lung disease always be diagnosed by x-ray examination?

For all practical purposes, yes. Sometimes it is necessary to have repeated examination or films taken from several angles before a definite diagnosis can be made.

What harm can result from tobacco smoking?

Aside from the local irritating effects of the smoke on the membranes of the nose, throat, larynx, bronchial tubes, and lung tissues, there is a great deal of evidence that cigarette smoking predisposes toward development of cancer of the lung.

What is the significance of a chronic cough with expectoration of mucus?

It is indicative of irritation or inflammation in the larynx, windpipe, or bronchial tubes, and merits medical investigation.

X-ray of Normal Lungs. It is good practice for all adults, especially those living in crowded cities, to have a chest x-ray at least once a year. Such x-rays may discover tuberculosis, lung tumors, or any other abnormalities in the earliest stages of development.

Should one swallow the mucus he has coughed up or should he spit it out?

It should not be swallowed as it may upset digestive processes. Also, if such material contains tuberculosis germs, it may cause an intestinal infection. Sputum should be expectorated into tissues or receptacles which can be discarded without spreading germs.

What is the main significance of coughing up blood?

When a patient coughs up blood it is most important to determine whether he has tuberculosis or a tumor of the lung. These are the most important conditions that cause coughing up of blood, but any small break in a blood vessel in the throat, larynx, or bronchial tubes can cause blood spitting. Thus, this symptom does not necessarily mean that tuberculosis or cancer exists.

Can breathing of excessively hot air hurt the lungs?

The lining of the bronchial tubes and lungs can be burned seriously when hot steam is inhaled. This occurs occasionally in industrial accidents.

Can exposure to extremely cold air hurt the lungs?

Deep breathing of extremely cold air, as in the polar regions or at very high altitudes, can produce "frostbite" of the lining of the windpipe and bronchial tubes, with subsequent development of pneumonia.

Can one live a normal life with one lung removed or non-functioning?

Yes, if the remaining lung has adequate function. Restriction of activity would depend upon the degree of impairment of the remaining lung.

ATELECTASIS

What is atelectasis?

A condition in which the lung tissue is collapsed and contains no air.

What causes atelectasis?

Obstruction of a bronchial tube.

What types of atelectasis are there?

a. Those occurring at birth which are due either to a mucous plug in a bronchial tube or to a congenitally deformed and narrowed tube.
b. In later life, it may be caused by a blockage of a bronchus by mucus, pus, or blood. Also, foreign bodies, such as peanuts, meat, or other foods which have gone down the wrong way, may obstruct a bronchial tube and produce atelectasis.

What is massive atelectasis?

A postoperative complication in which there is a large amount of mucus plugging one of the main bronchial tubes. This may cause an entire lung to collapse.

What is the treatment for massive atelectasis?

A bronchoscope is passed into the trachea (windpipe) and the plug of mucus is sucked out with a suction apparatus.

Is massive atelectasis very common?

Not since anesthesia methods have improved so greatly. Anesthetists today keep the bronchial passages clear by sucking them out during and after the giving of anesthesia.

Is massive atelectasis a serious condition?

Yes. It is accompanied by high fever and marked shortness of breath. This may complicate the recovery of a patient who has just undergone surgery.

Is the present form of treatment effective in curing massive atelectasis?

Yes. The sucking out of the mucous plug and the giving of antibiotics will cure almost all cases of massive atelectasis.

Is it always necessary to have a bronchoscope passed to cure massive atelectasis?

No. Frequently, by stimulating deep breathing, the giving of oxygen, and stimulating the patient to cough, he can be helped to expel the mucous plug by himself.

EMPHYSEMA

What is emphysema?

A condition in which the lung tissue loses its elasticity and becomes overstretched. It is usually associated with partial obstruction of the bronchial tubes, so that air is trapped within the lung. Thus, air can get into the lungs readily but cannot get out easily. If this process continues, lung tissue becomes like an overstretched balloon.

In what condition is emphysema found most often?

Chronic bronchitis and asthma of long duration.

What are the symptoms of chronic emphysema?
   a. Increasing shortness of breath.
   b. Coughing.
   c. Gasping.
   d. Cyanosis (blueness of the skin, lips, and nails due to lack of oxygen).
   e. Decreased oxygen supply to the vital structures in the body.
   f. Eventual heart failure.

Does emphysema often progress to the above symptoms and to death?

No. Usually the symptoms are not so severe that they lead to heart failure and death.

Is there any satisfactory way to prevent emphysema?

Yes, by the prompt treatment of conditions such as bronchitis, asthma, sinus infections, and bronchiectasis. Also, by the avoidance of exposure to irritating factors, such as tobacco smoke, chemical fumes, and industrial dusts.

Does the overstretched lung found in emphysema ever rupture?

Yes. A cyst or blister on the surface of the lung, caused by emphysema, occasionally ruptures, causing spontaneous collapse of the lung.

What is another name for this sudden collapse of the lung?

Spontaneous pneumothorax.

SPONTANEOUS PNEUMOTHORAX

What are the symptoms of spontaneous pneumothorax or collapse of the lung?

There is a sudden and dramatic occurrence of chest pain, shortness of breath, and, occasionally, severe shock and collapse.

How does the physician make a diagnosis of spontaneous pneumothorax?

a. By noting the history of the onset.
b. By listening to the chest and noting the absence of breath sounds on that side.
c. By noting a resonant sound on tapping the chest with his fingers (percussion).
d. By taking an x-ray picture and discovering that the lung is collapsed.

What is the treatment for spontaneous pneumothorax?

Often, because of the sudden shock and severity of the symptoms, immediate hospitalization is necessary. Sometimes, when the air within the chest cavity accumulates and develops great tension (tension pneumothorax), a needle is inserted and the air is drawn off. This permits the collapsed lung to re-expand.

What other situations may produce spontaneous pneumothorax?

A perforation of the chest wall, such as a stab wound, gunshot wound, or a blast injury, etc. Also, a fractured rib may puncture the lung, allowing air to escape from it to the chest cavity, and thus causing the lung to collapse.

Is collapse of the lung ever a fatal condition?

Not if it occurs on one side only. However, some blast injuries or gunshot wounds may cause collapse of both lungs, and such a condition may lead to a fatality.

PNEUMONIA

What is pneumonia?

An infection, usually acute, of the air spaces and sacs of the lung.

What types of pneumonia are there?

They are usually classified as to cause, that is, as to whether they are caused by bacteria, viruses, fungus infection, or other types of germs.

What is lobar pneumonia, and how does it differ from bronchopneumonia?

Lobar pneumonia is an inflammation of an entire lobe or more than one lobe. It usually starts suddenly as a distinct illness, and causes, at its onset, chills and fever. Bronchopneumonia is an inflammation involving small patchy areas of lung tissue surrounding small bronchial tubes. It usually comes on more slowly than the lobar type and is seen most often as a complication of bronchitis, grippe, or influenza.

What is the most common variety of pneumonia seen today?

Pneumonia caused by a virus (virus pneumonia). Since the advent of the antibiotic drugs, the lobar type has become much less prevalent.

How do the antibiotics lessen the incidence of lobar pneumonia?

Since these drugs are so effective in the treatment of infections of the upper respiratory tract, they prevent the bacteria from gaining a foothold in the lungs.

What are the predisposing causes of pneumonia?

Undernourishment, fatigue, neglect of upper respiratory infections,

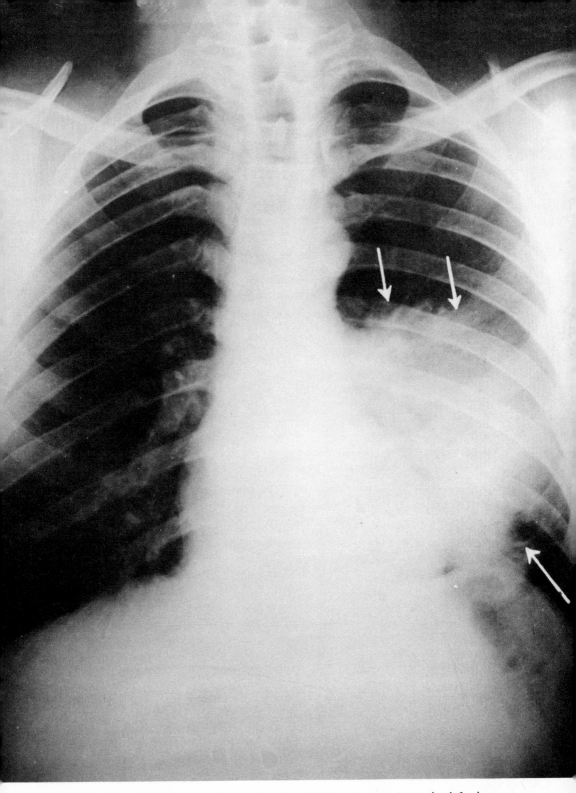

Lobar Pneumonia. This x-ray shows a lung with lobar pneumonia in the left chest. Note how the area within the field of the arrows is thickened and how air fails to enter the air sacs within the region infected by pneumonia. Through use of the antibiotic drugs, recovery from pneumonia is the general rule today, and this disease is no longer feared as it was years ago.

chronic alcoholism, and the aspiration of foreign material into the bronchial tubes.

What is the outlook for recovery from pneumonia?

Excellent. Years ago, almost one out of four people would die from a severe case of pneumonia. Today, a fatal termination is a great rarity.

How long does pneumonia last?

With adequate treatment, it usually can be cured within five to fourteen days.

How long must one stay in bed and remain at home after recovery from pneumonia?

At least two to three days after the temperature has returned to normal and after the antibiotic drugs have been discontinued.

Are there any unusual types of pneumonia which do not respond readily to treatment?

Yes; tularemic pneumonia, which is transmitted by rabbits; and psittacosis pneumonia (parrot fever), transmitted by birds.

What is aspiration pneumonia?

An inflammation of the lungs caused by the inhalation of a foreign substance, such as vomit, poisons, oily nose drops, or food particles which have gained access to the lung tissue through the bronchial tubes. This material often becomes secondarily infected by the growth of bacteria or viruses.

What is hypostatic pneumonia?

This type occurs in the course of certain chronic diseases, most often among elderly, weakened, bedridden patients. It is associated with a sluggish circulation within the lungs, which permits bacteria and viruses to gain a strong foothold.

Can hypostatic pneumonia be prevented?

In many cases, yes, by controlling the underlying disease and by frequent changes of the patient's position in bed. These patients should be gotten out of bed at the earliest possible time.

LUNG ABSCESS

(See section on Surgery of the Lungs in this Chapter.)

What is a lung abscess?

An area of pus formation within the lung.

What causes lung abscess?

It is usually caused by a blockage of a bronchial tube, with the development of infection beyond the point of obstruction. One of the most common causes is the aspiration of pus or infected mucus during an operation upon the nose, throat, or mouth.

Do lung abscesses ever occur without a preceding operation?

Occasionally.

How does one make a diagnosis of lung abscess?

a. The patient coughs up extremely foul-smelling pus.
b. There may be high fever, chills, and malaise during the early days of the illness.
c. There is a characteristic appearance of the lung on x-ray examination and the abscess cavity itself can often be plainly seen on the film.

Must lung abscess always be operated upon?

No.

PULMONARY EMBOLISM AND INFARCTION

What is pulmonary infarction?

The destruction of a portion of lung tissue due to interference with its blood supply.

What causes pulmonary infarction?

Usually an embolus (blood clot) which has traveled from another part of the body to a blood vessel within the lung. The blood vessel is obstructed by this blood clot and the tissue beyond it is said to have become infarcted.

Where do these emboli or blood clots usually arise?

From clotted blood in the deep veins of the legs or pelvic organs. These clots may form during the course of various disease processes or they may form as a complication of a surgical operation. Portions of the clot which break off and are carried through the bloodstream are termed emboli.

Does pulmonary infarction follow in all cases where there has been clotting of the veins in the legs or pelvic organs?

No. In the great majority of instances, the clot stays where it is in the veins of the legs or pelvis. It is only rarely that it breaks off and produces an embolus.

What are the symptoms of pulmonary infarction?

These vary with the size of the clot, the size of the vessel which has been plugged, and the suddenness of onset. There may be varying degrees of sharp chest pain, shortness of breath, cough, blood-streaked expectoration, and fever. In some cases, there may be severe shock or sudden death.

Will a pulmonary infarct show on x-ray examination?

Yes. In certain cases, it will show up as a haze on the lung film.

Is there any way to prevent pulmonary infarction in patients who have phlebitis (inflammation) in a leg vein?

Yes. In most instances it is advisable to use anticoagulant drugs (heparin or similar medications). These drugs keep the clot within the veins as small as possible and tend to prevent it from spreading or extending.

What is the outlook for recovery in pulmonary embolism?

The outlook is good in the majority of cases. Formerly, about 85 per cent of those affected had non-fatal embolism, while about 15 per cent of cases were fatal. Since the advent of the anticoagulant drugs, only about 1 per cent of cases end fatally.

How important is bed rest in pulmonary infarction?

Very important. Once a clot has formed, the patient must be kept at complete rest so that no further clot formation takes place and so that the chances of a piece breaking off are minimized.

DUST DISEASES
(*Pneumoconioses*)

Does exposure to dust always cause lung trouble?

No. Dust and fumes of many varieties may be inhaled over long periods of time without causing any disease of the lungs.

Which are the harmless dusts?

Dusts from iron welding and, to a great extent, carbon dusts from coal mining.

How does coal dust affect the lungs?

It produces no symptoms, even though the lungs of coal miners— and, as a matter of fact, all city dwellers—become black from the deposition of coal dust.

Which are the harmful dusts?

Those of silica (quartz), asbestos, talc, sugar cane, cotton fiber, and beryllium (dust from fluorescent light bulbs).

Which is the most serious dust disease?

Silicosis. This occurs from hard-coal mining, gold and lead mining, stone cutting and sand blasting, and the manufacture of certain abrasives.

How long must one be exposed to these irritants before symptoms are produced?

At least two years.

What are the symptoms of silicosis?

It causes progressive damage to lung tissue. This eventually leads to inflammation of the lungs; tuberculosis is a not infrequent eventual complication. There may be mild to severe shortness of breath,

815

chronic cough, and impairment of lung function. The endurance for work is markedly curtailed in serious cases.

How is the diagnosis of silicosis made?

By studying the patient's history, examining dust samples from the occupational site, and noting characteristic x-ray appearance of the lungs.

Can silicosis be prevented?

Yes, by providing healthful working conditions, and by providing masks and other protective equipment, such as vacuum blowers, etc.

Is there any treatment for silicosis?

No. Once scarring has occurred and lung function is impaired, there is no way of reversing the process. These patients must be guarded against further exposure to dust, or additional damage will result.

What is asbestosis?

A disease in which the inhalation of asbestos fibers causes lung damage. The symptoms are the same as those in silicosis.

What is byssinosis?

A disease of the lungs caused by inhaling cotton dust for a period of twenty years or longer. It is thought to be an allergic condition and produces cough and sputum, as in bronchitis.

SURGERY OF THE LUNGS

What are the various lung conditions for which surgery is sometimes required?

a. Infections.
b. Injuries to the lungs or chest cavity.
c. Cysts of the lungs.
d. Benign or malignant tumors of the lungs.

Are operations upon the lungs or chest cavity safe to perform?

Modern advances in surgical techniques and in anesthesia methods have made operations upon the chest practically as safe as those upon the abdomen.

How does a patient breathe when the chest cavity has been opened surgically?

Endotracheal anesthesia is utilized. By this method, oxygen can be supplied to the lungs without the necessity for active breathing by the patient. The endotracheal tube is inserted into the windpipe, and the anesthetist, by compressing the rubber breathing bag, controls the amount of gas which goes to the lungs.

INFECTIONS

Which types of lung infection may require surgery?

a. Lung abscess. The great majority of abscesses are now brought under control successfully with the antibiotics, but there are still a certain number of cases which will require surgical drainage. In former years, lung abscess was accompanied by a high mortality, but with modern methods of surgery and antibiotic therapy, practically all cases now get well.

b. Bronchiectasis. This is a condition in which the small bronchial tubes become widened and are partially destroyed. This makes them particularly susceptible to infection. When chronic infection sets in as a result of bronchiectasis, it is often necessary to operate and remove that portion of lung. This procedure, known as lobectomy, can be carried out safely and gives great promise of cure.

c. Empyema. This is a condition in which pus forms in the space between the lung and the chest wall (the pleural cavity). It was encountered often in bygone days as a complication of pneumonia. Today, it is a relatively rare condition, since pneumonia is controlled so effectively with antibiotics. However, when a case of pneumonia has been neglected or has been treated inadequately, empyema may develop. An incision into the chest cavity with drainage of the pus is the treatment of choice and will result in a cure in the great majority of cases.

d. Tuberculosis. (See Chapter 68, on Tuberculosis.) There are

817

many surgical procedures carried out for the cure of tuberculosis of the lung. These may include removal of an involved lobe or of an entire lung. Such procedures are called lobectomy or pneumonectomy. They are usually advocated only when the opposite lung is uninvolved in the tuberculous process. Thoracoplasty is advised in a certain number of cases. In this procedure, the ribs surrounding a tuberculous lobe of a lung are removed, thus allowing the chest cage to collapse and to permit the underlying lung to rest. Another procedure, known as a phrenic nerve crush, is occasionally recommended. This is carried out by making a small incision in the base of the neck, isolating the nerve, and crushing it with a clamp. The phrenic nerve supplies the diaphragm, and when it is crushed the diaphragm rises and becomes inactive, thus decreasing the size of the chest cavity and allowing the lung to collapse partially and to rest.

INJURIES TO THE LUNGS OR CHEST CAVITY

Are injuries to the lungs or chest cavity seen very often?

Yes, particularly in our mechanized society; accidents involving injuries to the chest wall and to the lungs are increasing at an alarming rate.

What are the most common injuries to the chest wall or lung?

a. Severe contusion of the chest cage.

b. Fractured ribs or fractured breastbone (sternum).

c. Laceration of a lung caused by the sharp edge of a broken rib being driven into the lung.

d. Air, blood, or both, in the pleural cavity surrounding a lung. This may come about as a result of lung puncture or as a result of a foreign body penetrating the chest wall.

e. Collapse of a lung secondary to spontaneous rupture or to hemorrhage.

f. Stab wounds or gunshot wounds of the chest.

Is it possible to save people who have received serious chest or lung injuries?

Yes. Contrary to general belief, the great majority of these people can be saved by proper surgical treatment.

What is the treatment for injuries to the chest cavity and lungs?

a. The first thing to treat is the shock which usually accompanies such injuries. Blood transfusions, inhalations of oxygen, and the giving of narcotics are a few of the immediate measures to be started.

b. If a gaping hole or sucking wound of the chest wall is present, the wound should be covered immediately so that air cannot enter the chest cavity from the outside. Tight bandaging of such a wound with gauze dressings and adhesive tape (or even with a torn shirt, if necessary) should be carried out as an emergency procedure whenever a sucking chest wound is encountered.

c. If hemorrhage from the lung into the chest cavity is severe, the chest cavity should be tapped by inserting a needle and withdrawing the blood. If the bleeding continues despite this procedure, then surgery should be performed and the bleeding brought under control by tying off the bleeding vessels, suturing the lung, or removing that part which is damaged.

d. Air may have collected around the lung (pneumothorax). This is withdrawn by inserting a needle or small rubber tube into the chest cavity and attaching it to underwater drainage. The lung will then expand and function again.

e. An extensively lacerated lung may have to be removed surgically.

Should people with severe lung injuries be transported lying down?

No. Injuries to the chest may create considerable difficulty in breathing and it is therefore best to transport these patients in a semi-sitting position.

CYSTS OF THE LUNGS

When are lung cysts encountered?

They are usually birth deformities and are characterized by thin-walled sacs filled with air or fluid. Some lung cysts produce no symptoms, while others will create pressure and cause collapse of surrounding lung tissue.

Do lung cysts ever become infected and form abscesses?

Yes. Others may burst and permit air to escape into the chest cavity.

What is the treatment for cysts of the lungs?

Those cysts which are causing symptoms should be removed surgically. Such an operation will involve removal of the cyst and surrounding lung tissue (segmental resection).

Are operations for removal of lung cysts successful?

Yes. The great majority of these patients make a complete recovery.

LUNG TUMORS

Are all lung tumors cancerous?

No. Benign tumors (adenomas of the lung) do occur, but, unfortunately, they are not encountered as frequently as the malignant growths.

What is the treatment for benign lung tumors?

Since it is almost always impossible to distinguish the benign from the malignant tumor preoperatively, the same surgical treatment is carried out for the non-cancerous growth as for the cancerous tumor.

Is lung cancer a common condition?

Yes. It is one of the most frequently encountered cancers in men.

Are cigarette smokers more prone to develop cancer of the lung than non-smokers?

This is a statistical fact, especially among men.

What are the early signs of lung cancer?

a. Persistent cough.
b. Chest pain.

c. Spitting of blood.

d. Characteristic findings of a shadow in the lung on x-ray examination.

Is there any way to tell if one is developing lung cancer?

The best protection is to undergo a yearly x-ray examination of the chest.

What is the treatment for cancer of the lung?

Surgical removal of the diseased portion of the lung (lobectomy), or removal of the entire lung (pneumonectomy).

Can a patient breathe normally after the removal of a lobe of the lung?

Yes, but his ability to engage in strenuous physical exercise is limited.

Can a patient live a normal life and breathe normally after the removal of an entire lung (pneumonectomy)?

Such people must refrain from strenuous physical exercise, but they can carry on most normal activity. Breathing is normal if they do not overexert themselves.

What fills in the empty space in the chest cavity after removal of a lobe of a lung or an entire lung?

The chest wall tends to collapse, the diaphragm ascends into the chest, and the empty space fills in with scar tissue.

Are the scars of operations upon the chest cavity or upon the lung very disfiguring?

There is a long twelve- to fourteen-inch incision coursing from the back to the front of the chest. However, this usually heals as a thin line and creates relatively little disfigurement.

Is the chest cavity badly deformed after the removal of a lobe of a lung or an entire lung?

No. When the patient is fully dressed, it is impossible to note that such a procedure has been carried out.

Is the chest markedly deformed after thoracoplasty (removal of several ribs)?

No. Such deformity is noticeable only when the patient is undressed.

Is anesthesia an important consideration in chest surgery?

Yes. It is vital to have good anesthesia during chest operations.

How long a hospital stay is necessary for removal of a lung or a portion of a lung?

Approximately two weeks.

Can patients get out of bed soon after major chest operations?

Yes, within two to three days.

What are the chances of ultimate cure following surgery for the following:

a. Tuberculosis: Excellent, with the great majority being cured.

b. Lung cysts: Excellent. Almost all cases will recover completely.

c. Lung tumors: For the benign tumors, the chances for permanent recovery are excellent. In cancer of the lung, more and more patients are being cured as the result of earlier diagnosis and improved operative techniques.

38 *The Male Organs*

THE PENIS, SCROTUM, AND TESTICLES
(See Chapter 55, on Prostate Gland.)

What is the structure of the penis?

It is composed of three tubular structures made of erectile tissue. Two of these are located on its upper aspect, and the third is on the lower aspect of the organ. The urethra, which transports the urine and seminal fluid, passes through one of these tubular structures. All three tubular structures, called corpora, are made up of spongy tissue and when filled with blood they become rigid, thus producing an erection. The head of the penis, or glans, is covered at birth by the foreskin. The latter structure is removed when circumcision is performed.

What is the function of the penis?

a. To transport urine.
b. To transport seminal fluid containing the sperm.

CIRCUMCISION

What is circumcision?

The removal of the foreskin.

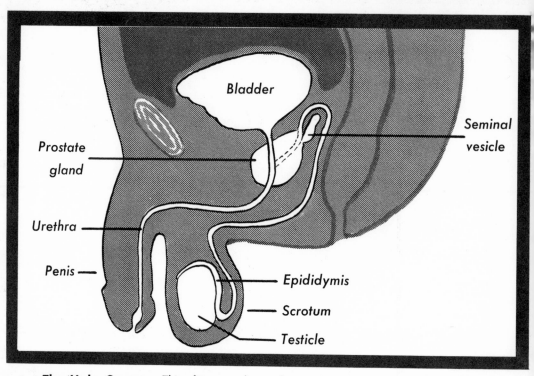

The Male Organs. This diagram shows the penis, prostate, seminal vesicles, and testicles. Sperm are manufactured in the testicles and are transmitted along the tube called the vas deferens and up into the seminal vesicles. The sperm are stored there and are emitted through the channel of the penis (urethra). Sperm is mixed with fluid secreted by the prostate gland before it is ejaculated.

Why is circumcision recommended universally?

Because it is almost certain insurance against the development of cancer of the penis, since this condition rarely occurs in circumcised males. It is also recommended because it is more hygienic and permits easier cleansing of the penis.

Is it true that women who are married to circumcised men are less likely to get cancer of the cervix or uterus?

Some investigators hold the theory, which seems to be borne out by recent statistics, that some of the material in an uncircumcised penis may act as an irritant when in contact with the cervix of certain women, and that, therefore, women who are married to circumcised men are less likely to develop cancer of the cervix.

When is the proper time to circumcise a newborn child?

Before he leaves the hospital, between the fifth and eighth day.

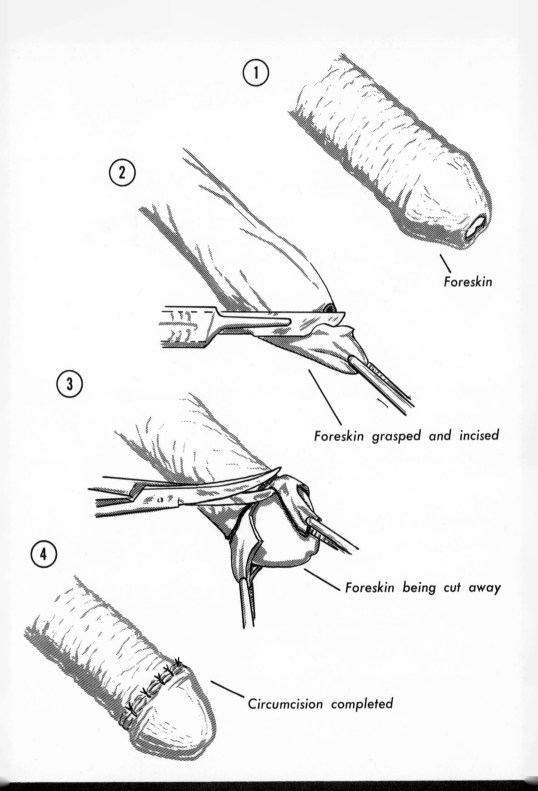

① Foreskin

② Foreskin grasped and incised

③ Foreskin being cut away

④ Circumcision completed

Circumcision. These diagrams show one method for performing circumcision. Most infants born today are submitted to circumcision because it is a safeguard against the development of cancer of the penis. Furthermore, a circumcised penis is much easier to

Is anesthesia necessary when performing circumcision?

No.

Is anesthesia necessary when circumcising older children or adults?

Yes.

How long a hospital stay is necessary when circumcising an older child or adult?

One to two days.

Are there any harmful effects from circumcision?

No.

TUMORS OF THE PENIS

Are malignant tumors of the penis common?

No, and as stated previously, they do not occur in circumcised males.

Where is cancer of the penis usually located?

Near the head of the penis, where it has the appearance of a protruding mass or a deep hard ulcer.

In what age group is cancer of the penis most likely to occur?

In middle and old age. It rarely occurs in youth.

How is the diagnosis of cancer of the penis made?

By taking a biopsy from the growth and submitting it to microscopic examination.

With what other condition can a cancer of the penis be confused?

One must distinguish a cancer from a venereal lesion such as a chancre.

Is cancer of the penis related to sexual activity?

No.

What is the treatment for cancer of the penis?

The best form of treatment is amputation of part or all of the penis, along with removal of the lymph glands in the groin which drain the penis. If the growth is small and is diagnosed early, it can be treated with the local application of radium or by a combination of local removal of the tumor plus radium application.

If the penis is amputated, how does urination take place?

A small stump of penis is left to permit this function to continue.

Can cancer of the penis be transmitted by sexual intercourse?

No.

THE SCROTUM AND TESTICLES

What is the scrotum or scrotal sac?

A semi-elastic muscular sac covered by skin, located beneath the penis. It is divided into two compartments, each of which contains a testicle, an epididymis, and a spermatic cord.

What is the composition and function of the testicle?

It is composed of a large number of tiny tubules known as the seminiferous tubules. It is here that sperm are produced. The testicle also contains cells which produce the male sex hormone, testosterone. The function of the testicle is to manufacture sperm and to allow them to be transported along the spermatic cord to the seminal vesicles. From the vesicles, the sperm are ejaculated during intercourse.

INJURIES TO THE TESTICLE

What is the treatment for an injury to the testicle?

The great majority of injuries, although extremely painful, are not serious and will heal by themselves. If the testicle is badly crushed or ruptured, it must be removed surgically.

Can an injury to a testicle lead to sterility?

Severe damage to one testicle may cause it to lose its ability to transmit sperm, but if the other testicle remains normal, sterility will not result.

Are injuries to both testicles very common?

No. Nature has a way of protecting these structures so that injury to both testicles is rather unusual.

TUMORS OF THE TESTICLE

What is the incidence of tumors of the testicle?

Malignant tumors of the testicle constitute about 5 per cent of all malignant growths seen in males.

Do tumors of the testicle occur more frequently in abnormally developed testicles and in undescended testicles?

Yes.

When are tumors of the testicle most likely to occur?

In the third, fourth, and fifth decades of life.

Are all tumors of the testicle malignant?

No, but malignant growths are much more frequent than benign growths.

How can one tell if a tumor of the testicle is present?

By the appearance of a slow, painless enlargement of the structure.

What causes tumors of the testicle?

The cause is unknown.

What is the treatment for these tumors?

Surgical removal should be carried out just as soon as the diagnosis is made. A radical procedure is performed if the growth is malignant. This will involve the removal of the lymph glands in the groin as well as the testicle.

Is x-ray treatment of value in treating tumors of the testicle?

Yes. After surgery has been performed, x-ray treatment is often employed to prevent spread of the tumor.

UNDESCENDED TESTICLE

What is an undescended testicle?

During the development of the embryo, the testicles are located in the abdomen. As the embryo grows, the testicles descend into the groin, and by the time the child is born, the testicles have reached the scrotal sac. Failure of such descent or incomplete descent is called undescended testicle (cryptorchidism). This may occur on one or both sides.

If there is an undescended testicle at birth, does it mean 'that the testicle will remain undescended?

Not necessarily. A certain number of testicles will descend during the first year of life or during adolescence.

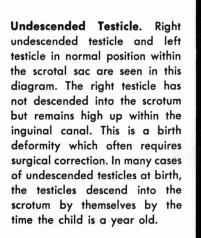

Undescended Testicle. Right undescended testicle and left testicle in normal position within the scrotal sac are seen in this diagram. The right testicle has not descended into the scrotum but remains high up within the inguinal canal. This is a birth deformity which often requires surgical correction. In many cases of undescended testicles at birth, the testicles descend into the scrotum by themselves by the time the child is a year old.

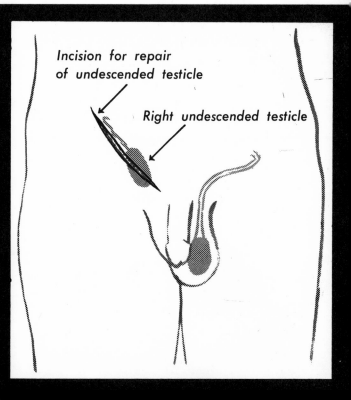

Incision for repair of undescended testicle

Right undescended testicle

What medical treatment can be given in order to encourage a testicle to descend into the scrotal sac?

Hormone injections will sometimes cause the testicle to grow and to descend into the scrotal sac.

Are undescended testicles often associated with the presence of a hernia?

Yes.

What is the best time to operate upon a child with an undescended testicle?

At nine to ten years of age.

Must surgery be performed on all children with undescended testicles?

Not if the testicle descends following a series of hormone injections.

What operation is carried out for undescended testicle?

There are many methods of performing this procedure (orchido-pexy). An incision three to five inches long is made in the groin and the testicle and cord are delivered into the wound. The cord is lengthened by cutting away all the extra fibrous tissue and adhesions which may be surrounding it. The testicle is then brought down into the scrotal sac where it is anchored in place with silk sutures.

Are operations for undescended testicle serious?

No. They are no more serious than a hernia operation.

How long a hospital stay is necessary for this procedure?

About five to seven days.

Will undescended testicles function normally when brought down into normal position?

Not always, since some of these glands are extremely small and underdeveloped. However, even if they fail to produce potent sperm, they will continue to secrete the important male sex hormone and thus maintain the male characteristics of the individual.

Are the results of operations for undescended testicles good?

Yes. The great majority of testicles can be brought down into the scrotal sac.

HYDROCELE

What is a hydrocele?

It is a collection of clear fluid within a membranous sac surrounding the testicle. It may also occur in the spermatic cord.

What is the cause of hydrocele?

The cause is unknown.

Does the presence of a hydrocele endanger the testicle?

No.

What is the treatment for hydrocele?

In small infants, hydroceles have a tendency to disappear by themselves. If they occur in older children or in adults, surgery is indicated.

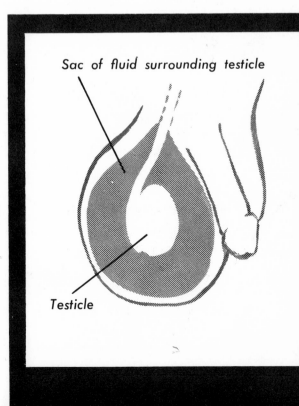

Sac of fluid surrounding testicle

Testicle

Hydrocele. This is a rather common condition in which the sac surrounding the testicle is filled with fluid. Many infants born with a hydrocele may require no treatment, as the fluid will absorb before the child is a year of age. However, when the hydrocele persists, surgery for its removal should be performed. The testicle is rarely damaged by the presence of a hydrocele.

What is the surgical treatment for hydrocele?

Through a small incision in the groin, the hydrocele sac is excised completely, or part of it is removed and the remainder turned inside out and sutured behind the testicle.

Are operations for hydrocele serious?

No. They are considered to be minor surgical procedures.

What are the results of surgery for hydrocele?

Cure of the condition.

Is there a non-surgical treatment for hydrocele?

Yes. The fluid within the hydrocele sac may be withdrawn through a needle and a solution may be injected to cause the walls of the sac to become sclerosed. This form of treatment is not as efficient as surgery and may occasionally result in infection.

Do hernias and hydroceles often occur together?

Yes, and when this does happen, both conditions should be corrected surgically.

TORSION (TWIST) OF THE TESTICLE

What is torsion of the testicle?

For some unexplained reason, in boys and young men, the spermatic cord and testicle may suddenly undergo a twist. This may be due to an excessively long cord, to a defect in its development, or to an injury.

What are the symptoms of torsion of the testicle?

There is sudden pain, marked tenderness, and swelling in the region of the testicle and along the cord. Nausea and vomiting may ensue. When the twist takes place, the blood supply to the testicle is shut off. Unless the condition is remedied promptly, the testicle may become gangrenous.

What is the treatment for torsion of the testicle?

Prompt surgery, with untwisting of the cord. In order to save the testicle, surgery should be performed within six to eight hours after onset. If, at operation, the testicle is found to be gangrenous and beyond salvage, it must be removed.

Is torsion of the testicle a serious condition?

It is serious in that it may lead to loss of one testicle, but not serious insofar as danger to life is concerned.

How long is the period of hospitalization for torsion of the testicle?

Five to six days.

INFECTION OF THE EPIDIDYMIS
(Epididymitis)

What is the epididymis?

It is a structure immediately adjacent and connected to the testicle. It is made up of innumerable tubules containing the sperm that have been manufactured by the testicle.

Are infections of the epididymis common?

Yes. In years gone by, when gonorrheal infection was so poorly controlled, many infections of this structure were seen. Today, however, antibiotic therapy has reduced the incidence of infection within the epididymis.

What are some of the causes other than gonorrhea for infections of the epididymis?

It is sometimes encountered after an operation upon the prostate gland or it may follow a cystoscopic examination with instrumentation and catheterization of the ureter.

How can one prevent infections of the epididymis?

The best way to prevent it is to tie off and cut the vas deferens (the tube connecting the epididymis with the seminal vesicles) before carrying out surgery upon the prostate.

What are the harmful effects of epididymitis?

In addition to being a very painful condition, with swelling, fever and extreme tenderness of the testicle, epididymitis is often followed by sterility if it involves both sides.

What is the treatment for acute epididymitis?

Treatment consists of bed rest, liberal fluid intake, the application of ice to the affected side, and the administration of antibiotics.

How long does the acute phase of epididymitis last?

About five to seven days, but the swelling may not subside for several weeks.

Is surgery ever necessary for epididymitis?

Yes, when an abscess has formed. This will require drainage.

Does acute epididymitis ever become chronic?

Yes. There are cases in which the infection subsides only partially and flares up from time to time.

What is the treatment for chronic or recurring epididymitis?

The surgical removal of the epididymis.

Is epididymitis ever caused by tuberculosis?

Yes, occasionally.

VARICOCELE

What is a varicocele?

A varicocele is a varicose involvement of those veins which accompany the spermatic cord.

What causes a varicocele?

It is thought to be a birth deformity. In 90 per cent of cases, it occurs on the left side.

Varicocele. This is a condition in which the veins coming from the testicle are varicosed. In most instances this condition requires no treatment. However, if there is pain in the area or if the varicocele is very large, surgical removal of the varicosities is indicated. This type of operation is not serious and results are uniformly good.

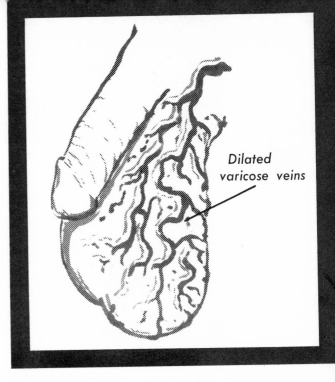

Dilated varicose veins

How is a diagnosis of varicocele made?

When the physician examines the scrotum, it will feel to him like a "bag of worms."

What symptoms are caused by varicocele?

Usually none, although there may be a dragging sensation and a feeling of vague discomfort at the side of the scrotum.

What is the treatment for varicocele?

Most varicoceles require no treatment. If they attain very large size, then surgery is performed, with the removal of some of the veins.

Are operations for varicocele serious?

No. They are carried out through a small incision in the side of the scrotum.

Is there any medical treatment for varicocele?

Yes. A well-fitting scrotal support may be worn.

Is fertility or potency affected by varicocele?

No, although an occasional patient with varicocele who is also infertile, will become fertile after surgical removal of the varicocele.

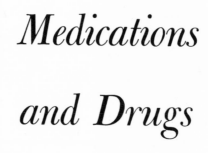

CHAPTER

39

Medications and Drugs

Is it safe for a patient to medicate himself without a doctor's advice?

It is absurd to assume that in every indisposition one should call the doctor before taking a simple medication such as a laxative or an aspirin tablet. However, intelligent people will realize that the physician should be consulted whenever unusual symptoms develop. In such situations, it is dangerous for people to medicate themselves.

If a physician has once recommended a medication, is it safe for the patient to take it again at a later date for what he considers to be a similar condition?

This should be done only upon the instructions of the physician. If there is any doubt at all, a brief telephone call may serve to avert a serious mistake.

Is it safe for someone to give a relative or friend a medication recommended for himself?

No. This has been the cause of many serious mistakes. Lay people

The Medicine Cabinet at Night. This photograph illustrates a most dangerous practice, reaching in the dark for a medication. Many serious accidents have resulted from people taking the wrong medicine. Everyone should make it a practice to turn on the light and read the label carefully before taking a medication.

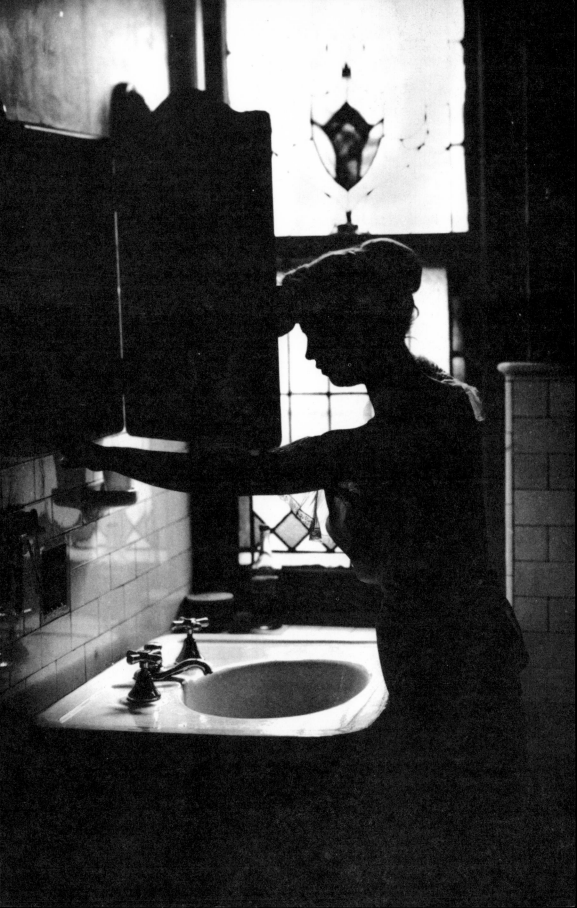

are not in a position to make an accurate diagnosis of another person's illness.

How can one tell if a drug or medicine is still effective or whether it has lost its potency?

Call your pharmacist or physician, if in doubt. Many prescriptions have labels which give an expiration date; look for this on the bottle.

Why is it that certain drugs can be bought directly across the counter while for others it is necessary to have a doctor's prescription?

Over-the-counter sale of drugs is regulated by federal, state, and local health authorities. The decision on these drugs is generally based on their possible toxic action as well as on the nature of the illness for which the drug is intended.

What controls are exercised by the government over the manufacture and sale of drugs?

The federal government sees to it, through its various agencies, that all medicines and drugs released for public consumption are properly manufactured, contain accurate information on their labels, and are based upon research which shows evidence that they are efficient for the illness for which they are prescribed.

How reliable are the various advertisements one sees and hears over radio, television, and in the newspapers about drugs and medicines?

It is safe to say that most manufacturers are a bit overenthusiastic concerning the value of their product. Some advertisements are cleverly misleading while still adhering to the letter of the law. On the whole, however, in America, one must say that advertisements maintain a rather high standard of accuracy. If they fail to live up to the law, the federal agency concerned is quick to prosecute.

How can one best safeguard against taking the wrong medicine or drug?

Whenever in doubt about a medication, call your pharmacist or family doctor on the telephone.

Should one ever take a drug or medicine when the label has come off or is difficult to read?

No. It is much safer to throw away the medicine than to take it without being certain of what it is. A safe rule is to always read every label twice before taking medication.

What medicines and drugs should be kept in the home medicine cabinet?

Unless one lives in a very rural district, it is not wise to keep too many medications at home. First-aid materials, a mild antiseptic, aspirin, and a few other similar medications are all that should be kept in the home.

What medicines and drugs are particularly dangerous to have around the house?

All medications and drugs are particularly dangerous to small children, who may overdose themselves. Even a laxative can be dangerous if taken in large quantities by a small child. All medications should be kept well out of the reach of small children, especially insecticides, lyes, and chemicals of any type, including alcoholic beverages.

What makes a drug habit forming?

a. The inherent character of the drug.
b. The personality of the individual who takes the drug.
c. Any drug which relieves discomfort and produces a pleasant state of mind or body is potentially habit forming.

Is there a difference between a habit-forming drug and a drug to which one has become addicted?

Yes. Drug addiction produces a physical and mental dependency upon the substance. Withdrawal of such a drug produces extremely intense physical, physiological and emotional disturbance. Withdrawal of a habit-forming drug may cause mild psychological and emotional distress, but rarely causes any physical symptomatology.

839

Is it true that the less medication a person takes, the better?

Yes. Medication should be taken only when necessary and the doctor's orders should be followed closely. It is just as bad to take too little medication when it is indicated as it is to take too much.

Is it common for people to develop resistance or immunity to the effect of various medicines after taking them for a prolonged period of time?

This tendency definitely exists with certain drugs. For instance, certain bacteria will develop resistance to penicillin and other antibiotics. Also, increased tolerance or resistance to the effect of certain pain-relieving drugs or narcotics or sleeping pills sometimes occurs. However, most medications continue to exercise their therapeutic properties when used properly over prolonged periods of time.

Can true drug addiction ever be cured?

Yes, though it is admittedly a most trying and difficult procedure.

Are there satisfactory measures to cure and control overdoses of medications and drugs?

There is a method of treating overdosages of all medications and drugs. The most important point to remember is not to delay one moment in getting medical help. Also, it is important to try to induce vomiting as soon as possible.

Why is it that so many physicians refuse to renew a prescription but will insist upon a return visit?

a. To check on the progress of the patient and the effect of the medication.
b. To make certain that there are no new complications.
c. To reaffirm or to alter a questionable diagnosis.
d. To alter dosage or to change the medication.
e. Certain medications are effective for only short periods and should not be taken for prolonged periods of time.

Should pregnant women be especially careful about the medicines or drugs they take?

Yes, particularly during the first few weeks of pregnancy as medications beneficial to the mother may have serious, harmful effects upon the embryo.

Is it harmful, at any time, to take a medication for too long a period?

Yes. Certain medications, while effective and harmless for short periods of time, will cause toxic symptoms if taken for too long a period. Consult your physician.

ANTIBIOTIC DRUGS

What are the antibiotics?

Antibiotics are chemical substances produced by living micro-organisms such as bacteria or fungi. They are used medically to combat disease produced by other bacteria or viruses.

What are some of the most widely used antibiotics?

Penicillin, streptomycin, tetracyclin, chloramphenicol, novobiocin, etc. New antibiotics of extreme value are being discovered every year.

How effective are the antibiotics?

Millions of lives have been saved since the antibiotics have been discovered. Pneumonia, streptococcal, staphylococcal, gonococcal, syphilitic, and other infections have been cured by the judicious use of the antibiotics.

Does one tend to develop resistance to the antibiotics?

The patient does not develop resistance to the antibiotics, but unfortunately many bacteria do develop resistance. Antibiotics should therefore be used wisely and sparingly.

Are antibiotics helpful in the treatment of tumors or cancer?

At the present time, there are no known cures from the use of the antibiotics in the treatment of tumors or cancer. However, extremely encouraging research along this line is at present in progress.

Is allergy to the antibiotics common?

Yes. However, a patient may be allergic to one antibiotic and not to others. Thus, allergic patients can be treated successfully with one or another of these wonder drugs.

Is it safe for someone to medicate himself with the antibiotics?

No! Antibiotics should be taken only upon a doctor's prescription, because self-medication may lead to unnecessary development of allergies to the antibiotics or to the development of resistance of certain organisms within the body to the antibiotics.

Are harmful effects ever seen from an allergy to, or overdose of, antibiotics?

Occasionally. The allergic reactions may be most severe and may show themselves by skin rashes, bleeding tendencies, and hives. Antibiotics may cause serious damage to the kidneys, the bone marrow, the nervous system, or to the gastro-intestinal tract. As in all other potent medications, their usage should be outlined and controlled under a physician's direction.

Should prescriptions always be obtained before taking antibiotics?

Yes.

Are antibiotics effective against the common cold or grippe?

Not at all.

SULFA DRUGS
(*Sulfonamides*)

What are the sulfa drugs?

A specific class of chemical substances, synthetically manufactured, which are effective in the treatment of a wide variety of bacterial and viral diseases. They are often used interchangeably or in conjunction with the antibiotics.

How effective are the sulfa drugs in the treatment of infection?

The sulfa drugs are one of the greatest advances achieved in medical therapy over the past twenty years. In certain types of infection, they are even more effective than the antibiotics.

Do patients ever develop immunity or resistance to the sulfa drugs?

Here again, the patients themselves do not develop a resistance or immunity to sulfa drugs, but certain bacteria do become resistant. Reactions of an unfavorable nature are quite uncommon when using the more modern sulfa drugs.

Is it safe to medicate oneself with the sulfa drugs?

No. These medications are powerful and should be taken only upon a doctor's prescription.

Is it necessary to drink large quantities of fluids when taking the sulfa drugs?

Yes, as this will prevent crystals from precipitating in the kidneys and in the urine. However, recent improvements in the structure of the sulfa drugs has minimized this complication.

Do the sulfa drugs ever adversely affect the blood-forming structures?

This is now a rare occurrence. However, if taken over a prolonged period of time, it is wise to have a routine blood count taken. Also, it is wise to have the urine examined to note the appearance of crystals or blood cells.

Are antibiotics more effective than the sulfa drugs in combatting infection?

Only in certain types of infections. Conversely, there are many types of infections for which the sulfa drugs are more effective than the antibiotics.

Are the antibiotics safer to take than the sulfa drugs?

No.

843

PAIN-RELIEVING DRUGS
(*Analgesics*)

What are the common analgesic medications?

The most commonly used analgesics are salicylates, that is, aspirin and related medications.

How effective are the analgesics in relieving pain?

Aspirin and aspirin-like medications are usually very effective means for relieving pain. They are relatively mild in action and are of great usefulness. However, they are relatively ineffective against the more serious causes of pain, such as kidney colic, ulcer pain, etc.

Is it safe to medicate oneself with the analgesics?

Prescriptions are not usually required for the purchase of most mild analgesic medications. Some self-medication is permissible, provided it is done intelligently. In other words, their usage for temporary minor aches and pains is permissible. However, they should not be used for conditions which are severe and which continue over a prolonged period of time.

Is there any harm in taking analgesics over a period of many weeks or months?

Any condition which requires an analgesic to be taken for weeks or months, warrants examination by a physician.

For what common conditions are the analgesics usually prescribed?

Minor muscle aches and pains, neuralgias, functional headaches, arthritis, menstrual cramps, and other conditions not requiring narcotics for relief.

Is aspirin habit forming?

No.

Does one develop an allergy or an immunity to the analgesic medications?

Allergy to analgesics does occur and is frequently seen. However, these medications are quite remarkable in that long-term, frequent use is not commonly associated with loss of efficacy of the drug.

Is it important to take the correct dosage of aspirin or other analgesic drugs?

Definitely, yes. Incorrect dosage may be dangerous if too high, or ineffectual if too low. Dosage will always vary according to the age and weight of the patient.

Are analgesics ever dangerous to take?

Yes, when a patient is allergic to them. Fatalities have been known from taking just one aspirin tablet. Also, the correct dosage is very important to determine in children, as a child may have undue sensitivity to this group of medications.

If a person is sensitive to one pain-relieving drug, is he likely to be sensitive to all of them?

Fortunately, no.

BARBITURATES

What are barbiturates?

They are medications which are commonly prescribed to allay nervous tension or for the purpose of inducing sleep.

How effective are the barbiturates in inducing sleep and relieving nervous tension?

Although there is great variability in the susceptibility to barbiturates, generally speaking they are effective in relieving nervous tension and in inducing sleep. It must be mentioned, however, that the underlying cause for the nervous tension and lack of sleep cannot be helped by taking barbiturates.

Should one medicate himself with barbiturates or should he take these drugs only upon a doctor's prescription?

Most emphatically, barbiturates should only be taken under doctor's orders, as they are potentially harmful drugs.

845

Is it safe to take barbiturates over a long period of time?

No, unless the physician permits this practice.

Are the barbiturates habit forming?

Yes. In certain people, they may even cause addiction.

Does one develop a resistance or immunity to barbiturates after taking them for a period of many months?

Yes. To achieve the same effect from barbiturates, users tend to require larger and larger dosages.

What harm can result from an overdose of barbiturates?

Marked overdose of these medications may cause coma or death.

For what conditions are the barbiturates commonly prescribed?

Nervous tension, irritability, convulsive states such as epilepsy, motion sickness, insomnia, overstimulated states, high blood pressure, etc.

Are there drugs, other than the barbiturates, which are effective for sedation?

Yes. The bromides, chloral hydrate, and some of the newer non-barbiturate drugs have been found to be effective.

Are there instances when the above-named drugs are preferable to the barbiturates?

This will depend upon the individual patient's response and the particular preference of the prescribing physician.

TRANQUILIZERS

What are the tranquilizer medications?

These are chemicals which are supposed to have the peculiar property of allaying tension and anxiety without causing drowsiness or in any other way adversely affecting mental processes.

Can one buy the tranquilizer drugs across the counter or should a doctor's prescription be obtained?

According to law, these drugs should be prescribed by a physician. However, in many areas this regulation is not strictly observed.

Is it safe to medicate oneself with tranquilizing drugs?

Definitely not. People who feel they need a tranquilizer, need medical attention first. The decision to prescribe these drugs should come from the physician and should not originate with the patient.

Does one ever develop an allergy or resistance to tranquilizers?

Severe allergic and toxic reactions to these drugs have been reported. It is too early to say whether resistance develops, but there are indications that this may be so.

How effective are the tranquilizers in calming the nerves?

Early reports indicate enthusiastic response. However, longer and more objective observation is required before a final evaluation of their effectiveness can be made.

Is there any harm in taking the tranquilizer drugs over a period of months or years?

It is too early to make such an evaluation. Early indications are that taking these drugs over a period of years may well lead to harmful consequences in certain people.

Can an overdose of tranquilizing drugs be dangerous?

Yes. Severe toxic reactions have been noted with large overdoses of these medications.

Are the tranquilizers a good substitute for the narcotics or barbiturates or the analgesics?

Tranquilizers should not be considered in the nature of a "substitute" for any of these other types of drugs, although there is often an overlap in their areas of usage.

NARCOTICS

For what purpose are the narcotics prescribed?

They are the most potent pain killers and are prescribed only in situations where pain is intolerable or excruciating.

Can narcotic drugs be obtained directly, or is it necessary to have a doctor's prescription.

A doctor's prescription is mandatory.

What advantages do the narcotics have over the pain-relieving drugs?

Narcotics are many, many times more potent than the analgesic drugs.

Should narcotics ever be used in place of the barbiturates or tranquilizers in order to produce sleep or relieve nervous tension?

No! Narcotics should never be used in the treatment of insomnia or nervous tension.

How can one tell if he is becoming addicted to a narcotic?

The patient will experience an intense emotional craving for the narcotic as well as extremely unpleasant physical symptoms if the drug is not taken.

Does one ever develop immunity or resistance to the effects of narcotics?

One does not become truly resistant to narcotics, but frequent usage may lead to the necessity of ever increasing dosages in order to produce the same effect.

How quickly does one become addicted to some of the more powerful narcotics?

It usually takes at least several weeks of repeated use to induce addiction. However, extremely susceptible people have been known to become addicted after only a few doses of a drug.

Is there a cure for narcotic addiction?

Yes, but it usually requires a great deal of effort and perseverance.

LAXATIVES
(*Purgatives*)

Is it safe to take laxatives?

In most cases, it is quite safe to take laxatives to relieve occasional or chronic constipation. This does not mean that frequent and repeated use is admissible.

When should one *not* take laxatives?

a. When there is acute abdominal pain.
b. When there has been progressively increasing constipation which appears to respond less and less to laxatives.
c. When there are symptoms such as chest pain, headache, or other signs not related to the bowel.
d. When there is evidence of bleeding from the intestinal tract, such as bloody stools or black stools.

When should one consult his physician concerning the taking of laxatives?

a. In all of the above instances, or in any other situation where there is doubt as to the propriety of taking a laxative.
b. When one finds that he cannot get along without the repeated use of laxatives.

Do laxatives tend to be habit forming?

Definitely, yes.

Do laxatives tend to lose their effectiveness if taken over a period of months or years?

Yes.

Can permanent damage be done to the bowels by prolonged usage of laxatives?

Yes. The bowels may lose some of their ability to function naturally. In other instances, the frequent taking of laxatives may irritate the lining of the bowel and lead to certain types of colitis.

How can one break the laxative habit?

This is most difficult, and will require gradual weaning from the use of laxatives and a substitution of new habits. Foods plentiful in bulk and roughage should be taken. Most important of all, the individual must establish a fixed daily routine for bowel movements. It is important to consult your physician to make sure that no underlying disease is the cause for the chronic constipation.

Are there any adequate substitutes for laxatives?

Yes. There are several preparations which are not true laxatives but which form bulk and moisture in the intestinal tract.

Can overdose of laxatives ever be dangerous?

Yes. Certain of the ingredients in some of the laxatives can cause serious toxic reaction.

WEIGHT-REDUCING DRUGS

What are some of the common weight-reducing drugs?

There are no true weight-reducing drugs but merely drugs which tend to make the patient lose his appetite. The most commonly used drugs are in the amphetamine group.

Is it safe to take weight-reducing drugs without a doctor's prescription?

No. Do not take another person's prescription simply because it works for him; it may cause serious injury to *you.*

Are the bulk-forming drugs safe to take in order to reduce appetite?

There are certain medications which form large bulk within the stomach and tend to make the patient lose his appetite. However, these drugs are not without danger and should only be taken when prescribed by a physician, as they sometimes cause intestinal disorders.

Can weight-reducing drugs be taken over a prolonged period of time if the patient *is* supervised by a physician?

Yes.

Is there a tendency for the effectiveness of the weight-reducing drugs to wear off if the drug has been taken over a prolonged period of time?

Yes.

Are there any safe weight-reducing drugs which will permit the patient to eat a normal, full diet?

No. Unless the calorie intake is decreased, the patient will not lose weight.

HORMONES

What are hormones?

They are the secretions of the endocrine glands.
Hormones are chemicals which are secreted into the bloodstream by these glands and which affect the body mechanism as a whole.

What are the common hormones within the body?

a. Pituitary hormone, secreted by the pituitary gland.
b. Thyroid hormone, secreted by the thyroid gland.
c. Parathyroid substance, secreted by the parathyroid gland.
d. Adrenal hormones, including cortisone and adrenalin, secreted by the adrenal gland.
e. Ovarian hormones, secreted by the ovaries.
f. Testicular hormones, secreted by the testicles.

Can hormones be manufactured artificially so that they can replace a deficiency in one's own body?

Many, but not all, hormones can now be synthesized chemically.

Should hormones ever be taken by a patient without a doctor's prescription?

No. Great harm may be done by improper usage of these powerful substances.

How effective are the hormones in treating glandular deficiencies?

This varies markedly with the condition for which they are being used. Suffice it to say that there are numerous conditions, both glandular and non-glandular, in which hormones have great therapeutic value.

What harm can result from taking hormones over a prolonged period of time without proper supervision?

If taken without proper supervision, hormones can cause severe imbalance in the chemistry of the body and may lead to serious illness and disorders. Hormones should only be taken under adequate supervision of a physician, who will make frequent tests to see if proper dosages are being given.

Can the indiscriminate taking of hormones lead to cancer development in an organ?

To date, there is no conclusive proof that an overdose of hormones can produce cancer, but it is conceded that certain hormones may well speed the growth and spread of latent malignancy. Thus, if a cancerous tendency exists, hormones must be given very cautiously.

Do people ever develop allergies to hormones?

Yes; this occasionally takes place.

Why is it that some hormones can be given in tablet form while others must be injected?

Some hormones are either destroyed by the digestive juices or are not properly absorbed in the intestinal tract. Such hormones must therefore be given by injection.

Are hormones of value in the treatment of glandular insufficiency?

Yes. Certain hormones, such as thyroid, ovarian, testicular, etc., are of great value if properly utilized in the treatment of inactivity of the endocrine glands.

What is cortisone?

This is a substance naturally produced by the adrenal glands. It belongs to the family of substances known as hormones.

What is ACTH?

This is an abbreviation for the term adrenocorticotrophic hormone. It is one of the substances normally secreted by the pituitary gland. Its function is to stimulate the adrenal gland to produce cortisone and cortisone-like chemicals.

What conditions are ACTH and cortisone used to treat?

In recent years, it has been discovered that both ACTH and cortisone are very effective in relieving a wide variety of diseases of inflammatory, allergic, or unknown origin. Some of the most common uses have been in various types of arthritis, rheumatic fever, allergies, sensitivities, lupus, nephrosis, etc.

Are ACTH and cortisone curative when used for the above conditions?

No. They merely alleviate the conditions, but it is felt that they may forestall physical damage due to the active process of certain diseases for which they are used.

Are ACTH and cortisone used in all cases of arthritis?

No. They are to be used only in severe cases of certain types of arthritis or in those that fail to respond to other forms of medication.

Which hormone is more effective, ACTH or cortisone?

They are usually equally effective. However, some physicians appear to show preference for one over the other in certain conditions. They are often used in an alternate fashion.

Is one of these substances safer than the other?

No.

Can ACTH or cortisone be harmful if given in excess quantity?

Yes.

Should ACTH and cortisone be given only under the supervision of a physician?

Yes! Improper and unsupervised use may cause serious damage.

Does the effect of these drugs continue after they have been stopped?

Unfortunately, most of the beneficial effects of these drugs are completely lost after they have been discontinued.

How is ACTH given?

ACTH is only effective when given by injection.

How is cortisone given?

Cortisone and some of the related drugs are effective when given either by mouth or by injection.

STIMULATING DRUGS

What is a stimulating drug?

One that acts upon the higher nervous system to eliminate a sense of physical or emotional fatigue. They are also used to counteract depression, drowsiness, and other lethargic states.

What are the more commonly used stimulating drugs?

Benzedrine, Dexedrine, ephedrine and caffeine.

For what purposes are stimulating drugs used?

a. To counteract mild depression.
b. To counteract certain neurological abnormalities.
c. To serve as a mild booster in patients who are unduly fatigued.
d. To counteract barbiturates or the toxicity of other depressant drugs.

Do stimulating drugs tend to lose their usefulness if they are taken over a prolonged period of time?

Usually not.

Can one develop an addiction or habituation to the taking of stimulating drugs?

True addiction to this group of drugs is uncommon. Habituation, however, frequently does occur.

Are stimulating drugs dangerous to take by oneself?

Most of these medications are potent chemicals and should be taken only upon a doctor's prescription.

Is it harmful to take an overdose of the stimulating drugs?

Definitely, yes.

Is caffeine a stimulant?

Yes.

Can the caffeine in coffee cause insomnia?

In those people who are sensitive to its use, insomnia can definitely be caused by a cup or two of coffee in the evening.

Does tea contain caffeine?

Yes. A cup of tea has approximately the same amount of caffeine as a cup of coffee.

Does cocoa contain caffeine?

Only in insignificant quantities.

Is alcohol a true stimulant?

No. On the contrary, alcohol is a depressant.

VENEREAL DISEASE DRUGS

(See Chapter 71, on Venereal Disease.)

VITAMINS

(See Chapter 72, on Vitamins.)

40

Mental Health and Disease

What is psychiatry?

It is that branch of medicine which is devoted to the study and treatment of conditions which affect the mind, human behavior, and the emotions. Some of these disorders are associated with structural changes within the brain, so that the fields of psychiatry and neurology often overlap.

What is psychology?

It is a branch of biology concerned with the study of all phases of behavior and conscious life.

What is a psychologist?

A specially trained person, usually not a physician, whose efforts are devoted either to teaching and research in the field of psychology or to clinical work in testing intelligence and applying psychological tests.

What is the incidence of mental disease?

Emotional disability represents the nation's foremost health problem. The extent of mental illness in its milder forms cannot be estimated, because one cannot draw a sharp line between the mild emotional disturbances of normal living and neuroses. It is said that about one of every ten people can expect to become mentally ill at some time.

Mental illness now occupies half the hospital beds of the country and the number is increasing every year.

Although the incidence is increasing year by year, the recovery rate is also increasing rapidly.

What are emotions?

Emotions are normal components of human experience representing the feelings people have in and about various situations which may confront them. They represent the responses in feeling to one's experiences. Fear, love, hate, anger, etc., are examples.

What are neuroses?

Neuroses represent patterns of emotional reaction which are inappropriate, excessive, and abnormal. Neurotic reactions are those which exceed ordinary emotional responses. They represent behavior in which the emotions get out of hand and dominate people. These reactions are often brought out by circumstances which disturb the patient in some way, and we speak of these circumstances as being "emotionally charged." Often, they are determined by unrecognized or unconscious motives—called conflicts—which are beyond the control of the individual. They include such phenomena as anxiety, emotional storms, irritability, compulsive phenomena, phobias, and certain types of depression, especially the reactive types. In a real sense they represent immature responses to situations.

How are neuroses treated?

By various forms of psychotherapy carried out by properly trained personnel, usually psychiatrists.

What is meant by the term psychoneurosis?

It is the same as neurosis.

What is the difference between a neurosis and a psychosis?

A neurosis is generally an emotional reaction of which the patient is fully aware. A psychosis is a form of mental illness in which the patient is in some manner disorganized and out of contact with reality.

857

Do neuroses often turn into psychoses?

No. This is a common misconception.

What is an anxiety neurosis?

A form of emotional disorder characterized by morbid anxiety. Such patients are tense, irritable, apprehensive, and explosive in reaction to situations. Sleep is apt to be poor. These patients also have certain physical manifestations, such as rapid pulse, palpitation of the heart, excessive sweating, trembling, dizziness, and headaches. There may be nausea and vomiting, or diarrhea.

Such symptoms may occur in relation to an obvious circumstance or problem, but at times the symptoms occur in attacks without any obvious cause and are accompanied by a sense of dread of impending disaster.

What is neurasthenia?

A form of neurosis in which excessive fatigue is present on slight exertion. It is often accompanied by hypochondria (undue concern about symptoms), loss of appetite, and loss of weight. There are likely to be additional complaints of neurotic origin, such as headaches, dizziness, insomnia, inability to concentrate, irritability, depression, etc. Many of these patients are actually suffering from a masked depression.

Can one have a nervous breakdown or become "insane" from overwork?

No.

Can one have a nervous breakdown or become "insane" because of great disappointment or tragedy in one's life?

Great tragedy can lead to depression of varying degree but rarely leads to a permanent mental illness.

What is insanity?

Insanity is a term of legal significance. It is no longer used by psychiatrists, except in a courtroom. It implies that a person is "insane" or "not of sound mind" and, as ordinarily applied, it means that the

858

person is not responsible for his actions. It is also employed as indi-cating that an individual is incapable of distinguishing between right and wrong. Many patients who are only mildly psychotic might not satisfy these criteria and might not be classed, legally, as being insane but would nonetheless be mentally sick.

What is meant by the term "nervous breakdown"?

This is a term used by lay people to refer to any emotional or mental disorder. It therefore has no clear or specific meaning.

Do reality situations play an important part in determining one's mental health?

Mental health depends less upon what actually happens to an indi-vidual than upon the individual's attitudes and how he accepts or faces reality problems.

What symptoms should be looked for to indicate that someone needs psychiatric help?

a. Frequent illnesses which are not clearly physical.
b. Prolonged or persistent complaints without proven disease or findings.
c. Frequent depression.
d. Irritability and uncontrolled temper.
e. Inability to carry on sustained work.
f. Persistent fatigue.
g. Too frequent conflict with one's associates.
h. Recurring anxiety and unfounded fears.
i. Persistent insomnia.
j. Unaccountable loss of appetite.

Will seeing a psychiatrist help to prevent a mental collapse?

Yes, in a great many instances.

Can one safely marry into a family in which a member is "insane"?

This depends upon the circumstances. In general, one can say yes. The fact that some other member is or was mentally ill has no bear-ing on the intended spouse if he or she is healthy.

What role does heredity play in mental disease?

It is uncertain how much heredity and environment contribute to mental disease. No doubt, some part of one's personality stems from his heredity, and this may contribute to the way in which a person will react in various situations and to various circumstances. However, it is felt that his environment and his experiences have the larger share in a person's development and make-up.

What part does sex play in determining mental health?

Adequate sex is part of mental health, although this may vary from one individual to another. Disturbances in one's attitudes toward sex, consciously or unconsciously, may cause emotional and mental disorder. On the other hand, emotional and mental illness frequently lead to sexual disturbances.

Does overindulgence in sex cause disturbance in mental health?

No.

Does lack of sex cause a disturbance in mental health?

Celibacy is practiced by a great many people without apparent emotional trouble. Thus, it cannot be said that lack of sex in itself impairs mental health. This is not, however, true for everyone. Many people do require some sexual experience and fulfillment. (Lack of sex may actually be the result of some emotional trouble, rather than the cause.)

Should one always take threats of suicide seriously?

Emphatically, yes! Patients frequently hide suicidal intentions and may appear casual in their expression of such thoughts. But the fact that the thought has been expressed is sufficient for it to be taken seriously. The intention may be stronger than the expression.

What is a compulsion neurosis?

Compulsion is part of an obsessive compulsive state. This is characterized by repetitive thoughts or actions which the patient is unable to overcome or control. (For instance, this is seen in people who wash their hands excessively, without logical reason.)

What is the significance of an abnormal attachment to a parent, as in the case of a "mama's boy"?

An abnormal attachment to a parent signifies an emotionally immature individual. Such a person is often unable to adjust adequately to life's situations.

What is meant by the Oedipus complex?

It is an unconscious attachment of a son for his mother coupled with jealousy of the father. This may result in feelings of guilt and emotional conflict.

What is meant by castration complex?

In psychoanalytic theory, it relates to anxiety about sex and a fear of being threatened with castration or deprivation of sexual organs.

What is claustrophobia?

It is a symptom often seen in patients with an anxiety neurosis. It is a fear of closed-in spaces such as elevators, tunnels, etc.

What is agoraphobia?

It is anxiety which develops in open spaces. It is part of an anxiety state.

Can fortune telling be harmful?

Yes. To an impressionable person subject to anxiety and superstition, it can be very disturbing.

Is there any value to hypnotism when performed by a psychiatrist?

Yes. Certain acute emotional disorders may be treated by hypnotism. Also, it may be helpful for gaining information which the patient finds difficult to transmit when in a conscious state.

Are there any objections to hypnotism being performed by people other than trained psychiatrists?

Yes. In certain susceptible and suggestible individuals, it can be harmful. It may even precipitate serious illness. Therefore, it should not be practiced without knowledge of the personality of the subject, and then only by a qualified psychiatrist.

Are sedatives harmful or dangerous for emotionally or mentally ill people?

Not in the doses ordinarily employed by doctors. Any danger would lie in taking large quantities, as for suicidal purposes. Therefore, potentially suicidal patients should not have access to more than small quantities of such medication.

Is it possible that a day will come when mental illness will be treated successfully by medication?

It is true that more and more drugs are being discovered which help the mentally sick. However, it is unlikely that a time will come when psychotherapy will be unnecessary.

What is insomnia?

The inability to sleep.

What are the causes of insomnia?

Where there is no symptom such as pain or bodily discomfort causing insomnia, it is caused by emotional disturbance. Thus, anxiety or worry or concern may retard sleep, or cause sleep to be fitful and restless.

Will the taking of sleeping pills cure insomnia?

No. Sleeping pills may afford sleep, but the cure will depend upon the alleviation of the underlying emotional disturbance.

Should people with insomnia seek psychiatric advice?

Yes, if the condition persists over a long period of time.

What is hysteria?

It is a fairly common form of emotional reaction in which the patient tends to act out his distress in exaggerated and dramatic form. The purpose of hysteria (consciously or unconsciously) is to attract attention and gain sympathy. These patients are generally very suggestible and may develop symptoms which have no basis in anatomical or medical fact. The illness is often precipitated by an event of dramatic quality, such as an accident, which is regarded by the patient as much worse than it actually is. Hysterical reactions are apt to come on abruptly. The patient becomes excited, noisy, and full of complaints, or he may be unduly quiet and indifferent to symptoms. He may appear to be in severe distress, much greater than can be accounted for by the real circumstances.

What are psychosomatic symptoms and diseases?

They are symptoms or diseases, usually of *physical* character, which are produced by *neurotic* (emotional) factors or in which neurotic factors play an important part. Such symptoms or diseases may arise in the stomach, where one might find hyperacidity (heartburn), indigestion, or even an ulcer. They may affect the bowel and cause a spastic condition, resulting either in constipation or diarrhea, in response to emotionally charged situations. When more persistent or more severe, psychosomatic disease may take the form of a true colitis, with formation of actual ulcers in the bowel wall. No organs of the body are immune to psychosomatic symptoms or disease, and they may manifest themselves as an allergy, a skin eruption, or other types of organic physical illness.

What are some of the more common diseases thought to be in the psychosomatic category?

Certain forms of hypertension (high blood pressure), peptic ulcer, and colitis, especially the spastic and mucous form and probably also the ulcerative type. This category also includes some of the so-called allergic conditions, such as asthma, eczema, hives, and various conditions in which itching is prominent, especially about the rectum and vagina. Also, hyperthyroidism (overactivity of the thyroid gland) and diabetes. Many forms of headache, including migraine, and certain forms of arthritis are considered by some physicians to be psychosomatic in origin.

Are emotional symptoms imaginary?

No, they are *real symptoms!* All too often, patients tend to think in physical terms and do not understand how a symptom can appear without a physical cause. They therefore conclude that if no physical basis is discovered, the symptoms are not real. Such symptoms are real even though they are engendered by emotion, and they may cause severe damage if not treated appropriately.

863

What is meant by organic disease of the nervous system?

Organic disease of the nervous system implies that there is structural damage or abnormal physical change. The term implies that the change is caused by a disease process, such as an infection or a tumor.

What is functional disease of the nervous system?

Functional disease refers to symptoms which are *not* due to abnormal changes in the tissues but to temporary physiological disturbances. Usually, these are the result of emotional factors which, through tension and various chemical (hormonal and endocrine) mechanisms, result in various symptoms.

When a person is nervous, agitated, or depressed, should he consult a psychiatrist?

Yes. Nervous and emotionally upset people can often be taken care of adequately by an intelligent, sensible, and informed doctor, but the true meaning and gravity of severe symptoms may not always be clear to a physician with limited psychiatric training. The trained and experienced psychiatrist may discover the serious implication of depression or of psychosis in one patient's preoccupations with bodily symptoms or in another's anxiety or confusion. Such insight may change the prospects and therapy to an important degree, or may suggest measures which may save life.

Will a patient be made worse by being placed in a mental institution?

No. Lay people often believe that a patient may be made worse by association with other mental patients. It is common practice in mental hospitals to separate various types and degrees of illness so that the less ill are not placed with the severely ill or violent patient. When symptoms are aggravated, it is likely to be the result of the natural progress of the illness.

Do people who enter mental institutions have much of a chance to be discharged as cured or improved?

Yes. A large proportion of the mentally ill get well. It is a common misconception that mental illness is always incurable!

Do mental institutions ever hold patients longer than they should?

No. This, too, is an erroneous idea. Mental institutions are most anxious to return as many of their patients as possible to normal life with their families and friends.

What is psychotherapy?

It is a form of treatment to help people with their emotional and mental problems. At a superficial level, in relation to the ordinary problems of everyday life, it may be carried out by intelligent and sympathetic people, such as one's friends and relatives; clerical people, such as ministers, rabbis, and priests; the family physician or lawyer. These people can often help with temporary and minor problems.

When problems are deeper and more persistent, when neuroses are present which are too much for the patient to manage himself, more skilled help is needed. This is provided by the trained and experienced psychotherapist. It is desirable that he be a physician because, so often, physical symptoms are present which must be assessed medically and because helpful medications require a doctor's specialized knowledge. However, there are not enough psychiatrists to meet present needs and non-medical (lay) psychologists, when adequately trained, have been serving successfully to fill the gap.

What are the aims of psychotherapy?

To help people to better understand themselves and to adjust to their difficulties and to help them to become more mature in dealing with their problems and with people with whom they come in contact. It is not the aim of psychotherapy to reform people, although part of its objective is the development of better values and standards.

Also, its aim is to treat and eradicate illness. To this purpose, the psychiatric therapist will use whatever means and methods are appropriate and have been known to be successful.

What is psychoanalysis?

This is a specialized form and technique of psychotherapy. Its aim is to bring enlightenment (insight) to a patient about the unconscious mechanisms underlying his personality and difficulties, hoping thereby to eliminate symptoms and improve the patient's reactions and responses. It operates solely through the patient, sometimes in a completely passive way. There are various schools with variations in theory, but the methods are much the same in all schools.

What is group therapy?

A method of psychiatric treatment in which a number of people, with similar problems or disturbances, are treated simultaneously as a group.

What are the objectives of group therapy?

Essentially the same as for individual therapy.

What advantage does group therapy afford over individual therapy?

a. It permits a larger number of people to be treated. This is very important today because of the marked shortage of well-trained psychiatrists.

b. This form of treatment is less expensive and therefore permits more people to avail themselves of help.

c. It makes available to the patient the experience of others so that he does not feel so alone in his illness.

What are the disadvantages of group therapy?

a. Treatment, and the attention of the psychotherapist, must be divided among several people.

b. It makes it more difficult for patients to express extremely personal problems.

c. The opportunity for individual therapy is lost.

How long does psychotherapy take?

This will depend upon the basic problems. These cannot be thoroughly determined until the psychiatrist breaks through the patient's defenses and is able to reach the inner thoughts which the patient himself may not be aware of. Hence, one cannot tell, in the beginning, how far one will have to go. Further, it will depend upon how frequently therapy takes place, and how determined the patient is to get well. Many patients are unaware of how deeply they are resisting the course of treatment. Intelligence is a factor, as is the age of the patient. Given an intelligent patient and one who is determined and persistent, in time much can be accomplished. Ordinarily, it is not a rapid procedure which can be accomplished in weeks. It requires months and often years to obtain good results.

Is psychotherapy expensive?

Yes. One must measure cost against the problem involved and against how emotionally expensive it is to retain the problems, the symptoms, and the difficulties. One cannot speak in absolute terms, but must consider the value received.

Is there any satisfactory surgical treatment for mental disease?

Until recently, a relatively simple brain operation, lobotomy, was advocated for certain types of mental illness, with occasional satisfactory results. The operation has, however, been largely abandoned since some of the newer medications have been found to produce similar results in selected cases.

What are psychoses?

The psychoses represent more severe disorders in which there is some degree of disorganized personality. The behavior has an aspect of unreality often unrelated to circumstances, and is often beyond the control of the individual. These diseases are classed as *mental* because there is some degree of irrationality or disorder of mind. They are apt to be characterized by bizarre and inappropriate behavior. Delusions and hallucinations may be present. The patients are often out of contact with their surroundings, and often are not accessible to rational and logical conversation.

Psychotics make up the large majority of patients in state mental institutions.

What are different forms of psychoses?

The psychoses include schizophrenia (dementia praecox), manic-depressive disorder and psychotic depression, paranoid disorders, involutional melancholia, and a group of organic diseases which may lead to psychoses. In the latter group are the senile psychoses,

psychoses due to some form of brain disease such as arteriosclerosis, brain tumors, syphilis, etc.

What is depression?

This is a form of reaction or disturbance characterized by lowering of the mood, or low spirits, or a gloomy outlook. Not only are the mood and spirits low, but general activity is also reduced. Patients suffering from depression lack pep and energy, lose interest in things, do not feel like doing anything or going anywhere, and wish to be left alone. They wish to remain at home. Their ordinary routine suffers and ordinary responsibilities are neglected. There is insomnia and loss of appetite, with consequent loss of weight. In a severe form, these patients become despondent, believe they cannot be helped, and neglect to seek help. Under such conditions, suicide is a distinct possibility and danger. Hence, experienced psychiatric help is urgently necessary and hospitalization is frequently desirable to protect the patient against himself. It is often better and wiser to have a patient safely in a hospital than constantly under a risk at home.

What is melancholia?

This is an older term formerly used in the same sense and meaning as depression.

Are there different forms of depression?

Yes. Depression is often part of a neurosis and may arise as a response to circumstances or problems. It is then called a reactive depression. The outlook for this is often good. In other cases, depression may be part of a mental disturbance or psychosis, usually limited in duration. Such episodes may be recurrent. Also, depression may be part of a manic-depressive or cyclic disorder.

What is involutional melancholia?

This is a form of depression occurring in later life. At times this represents recurrence of depression in a person who has had previous attacks of similar form. Therefore, it is not classified as a special type of depression. However, in some patients the depression is associated with considerable anxiety, agitation, and restlessness.

What is the treatment for depression?

First, one must take adequate safeguards against the risk of suicide if this tendency is present. When such thoughts are expressed they should not be ignored. Adequate safeguards should include constant supervision at all times. When the risk is great, hospitalization should be carried out.

Many psychiatrists believe that the best form of treatment is electro-shock therapy, which can be expected to benefit or break up a depression in 90 per cent of suitably selected patients. While some risk accompanies this form of treatment, it is not great when suitable safeguards are employed. If the risk is weighed against the suffering and risks of untreated depression, the balance is greatly in favor of shock treatment.

Within recent years, newer drugs have been discovered which appear to have a beneficial effect upon the depressed mood. In indicated cases, they can be used to good advantage, but certain forms of depression unfortunately fail to respond to these medications.

For what conditions is shock treatment indicated?

a. Severe depressions.

b. Manic states.

c. Dementia praecox (schizophrenia).

Are the results of shock treatment usually permanent?

The success of shock treatment may be permanent in certain cases, but this form of therapy should be followed up by intensive and prolonged psychotherapy in order to ensure lasting results.

Where can shock therapy be given?

a. In a psychiatrist's office.

b. In the clinic.

c. In the hospital.

What are manic-depressive reactions?

These are a group of psychotic disorders in which the patient may exhibit excitement (hence the term manic), incessant restlessness, and increase in all forms of activity, including speech. The mood is elevated and exhilarated. Such patients do not rest or sleep and are apt to wear themselves out if not checked. The symptoms vary in degree. Patients require some form of sedation, and if the symptoms are severe, they may require hospitalization and restraint.

On the other hand, the patients may be depressed, and they are then retarded in activity and depressed in spirits. Patients may remain in either phase for varying periods and then recover, or they may go from one phase into the other after a variable interval.

What is the outlook for manic-depressive psychosis?

Usually, the patient recovers from one episode after a varying interval of time, sometimes several months. He may remain well for some indeterminate time, only to become ill again. The new episode may follow the same pattern of illness as before, or the next phase may represent a swing in the opposite direction. Some patients remain well for long periods and have few episodes. Others may have many such attacks.

What is the treatment for manic-depressive reaction?

Electro-shock therapy is applicable to either phase of the disease and is usually quite effective. Psychotherapy is of some value in the lesser degree of sickness, not in the acute or severe forms. Appropriate and skilled nursing and management are important. Sedation is important in the excited phases. Certain stimulants may be helpful in the depressed phase. Psychotherapy should follow recovery from the episode, as it may be helpful in preventing a future recurrence.

Does change of life produce mental disease?

Not by itself, although glandular (endocrine) changes at this time may alter the general responsiveness of the person and add to her tenseness. Hence, this phase of life may produce various psychological stresses which may bring out inherent, latent trouble.

Does pregnancy or having a baby cause mental disease?

Not by itself, but having a baby is an emotional stress requiring adjustment to new responsibilities. It may, therefore, bring out emotional or mental reactions which have been dormant previously.

This period in a woman's life may require temporary emotional and psychotherapeutic support and help.

What is postpartum psychosis?

This is a form of mental disorder which develops in an exceedingly small number of women soon *after* confinement. It may take a variety of forms, including schizophrenia, manic state, depression, and states of anxiety or phobia resembling a neurosis. However, there is nothing in these disorders which is characteristic and they do not differ from similar patterns of disease occurring under other circumstances not related to pregnancy. Hence, this is not truly a postpartum disorder except in timing, and the confinement is only a precipitating factor.

What is schizophrenia?

This is a form of psychosis usually affecting younger people. It was formerly called dementia praecox. It is characterized by disturbances in thinking which are often bizarre, by impaired relation to reality, and by a split between thought content and the emotions. Thus, the patient may display no emotion in relation to his expressed ideas, or the emotions are out of keeping with his ideas. Hence, such patients are cold toward others. There is withdrawal from reality, often to a severe degree. In the early phase, these patients relate poorly to others and are often unable to hold a job for very long.

Can schizophrenia be treated?

Yes. Various physical forms of treatment have been of help, such as electro-shock and insulin shock treatment. Occupational and social therapy is helpful. Various newer medications have been useful, especially in the more disturbed cases. They have increased the number of patients discharged from hospitals. Recent research has had promising results and offers hope of even better modes of treatment in the near future.

What is the outlook in schizophrenia?

Often, it is poor; this condition, if untreated, is apt to progress. However, some patients recover from the acute forms and are said to have remissions (betterment). They may then be able to maintain themselves in a limited way, although they continue to have symptoms of mental illness to a milder degree, and may have difficulty in relation to other people.

Can treatment ever bring on a remission (betterment) in schizophrenia?

Yes.

What are paranoid reactions?

Mental disorders in which the patient has delusions of persecution. These delusions are such that he is convinced that certain people mean to do him harm. He distorts the slightest incident into proof of these delusions. Since these are delusions, the patient will not respond to reason. Laymen often refer to paranoia as a "persecution complex." There are several types of paranoid reactions, one of which is encountered in schizophrenia.

What is the outlook for a paranoid patient?

The condition may be temporary, as part of some transient, toxic, or organic disorder. At times, the disturbance may subside or remain stationary. More often, it is chronic and will progress until the patient requires admission to a hospital. The outlook in true paranoia is poor, inasmuch as psychotherapy cannot reach these unfortunate people.

What does I.Q. mean?

The letters stand for intelligence quotient. This is a figure derived from the ratio of *mental age,* as obtained by intelligence tests, to the *actual age* of the person. Average intelligence lies between 90 and 110 on this scale. Mental deficiency lies below this level.

What is mental deficiency?

Also known as mental retardation and feeble-mindedness, it refers to defective mental development present usually from birth or the early years of childhood. It implies a defect in understanding or comprehension and a handicap in learning. There are different grades or degrees of this, such as the idiot, imbecile, moron, or mentally retarded. Sometimes we speak of high-grade or low-grade deficiency. Usually there is some defect in the physical development of the brain. Hence, the disorder is essentially organic. Thus, there may be signs of other injury to the brain, such as paralysis, spasticity, or abnormal movement, or it may occasionally be associated with cerebral palsy. The head may be unusually small, with a correspondingly small brain. There may be hydrocephalus—a large head due to increased accumulation of fluid within the head and corresponding deterioration of brain substance.

What is Mongolism?

It is a variety of mental deficiency with a characteristic facial appearance. The cause is uncertain, but the majority of such cases occur when an older woman has a baby for the first time. These children have moderate retardation, are often docile, pleasant, and to an extent teachable. (See Chapter 29, on Infant and Childhood Diseases.)

What is idiocy?

This is the lowest form of mental development, easily recognizable early in life. The mental age never develops beyond two years. The I.Q. is below 25. Physical deformity may also be present, and convulsions are frequent. The idiot learns to talk very late and may never learn much speech. He can do very little for himself. He may be unable to care for himself or to dress and feed himself, and is likely to neglect himself. He requires considerable and constant supervision. He is likely to be irritable and destructive. Idiots occur about once in every 3,300 births.

What are imbeciles?

This form of mental deficiency is next above the level of idiocy. Symptoms are noted early in life. These patients develop late, learn very little speech, and are never able to take care of themselves. Speech is limited. Learning is poor, but they can be taught simple tasks. Mental age ranges from two to seven years, and the I.Q. falls between 25 and 50. Imbeciles occur about once in every 1,500 births.

Should idiots and imbeciles be institutionalized?

Many such children are much happier in an institution where specialized expert care can be given them. In considering placing such a child in an institution, parents should give primary consideration to the welfare of the child and the other members of the family.

What is a moron?

This term is applied to the group whose I.Q. ranges from 50 to 70. There may be delayed development, but the retardation in behavior may not be obvious. They look like other children and learn to walk and talk, and there may be no gross signs that these children are different from others. Only the fact that they may not get along as well as others in school work (which may have a variety of causes) and that they may have trouble with other children brings them to psychiatric attention. Only then is the retardation discovered by appropriate tests.

Into what category does a child with a 70 to 90 I.Q. fall?

This is the somewhat retarded child, who, with adequate training, can fit into society and live a useful life.

Is mental deficiency inherited?

In general, no. There are a few diseases in which mental deficiency is inherited, but these conditions are very rare and unimportant in the population at large. Most mental deficiency is accidental and occurs as a result of trouble at birth or follows acquired illness, infection, etc. It was once fashionable to regard most mental deficiency as inherited, but this was based on flimsy evidence which is no longer accepted.

What is an idiot savant?

Some individuals of very low mental development may reveal remarkable talent in one direction. Thus, they may disclose remarkable ability of calculation or memory in one area. Such an individual is called an "idiot savant."

What are the causes of mental deficiency?

a. Some mental deficiencies are due to hereditary disorders.

b. Some are due to illness in the mother while the child is developing, for example, German measles, especially when it occurs during the first three months of pregnancy.

c. It is sometimes due to difficult delivery of the baby or complications of pregnancy and the confinement.

d. It may be the result of injury or infection or other diseases affecting the brain in infancy or early childhood.

Is there any treatment for mental deficiency?

Mental deficiency cannot be cured or corrected, and people should not spend large sums of money on promises of cure. The patient requires appropriate care and management and direction so that his activities may be regulated to his capacities. Where emotional disturbance is prominent, suitable psychotherapy may help in the milder degrees of deficiency.

Are aptitude tests reliable?

Without an understanding of the personality of the individual and a knowledge of his intelligence, aptitude tests cannot tell a person what career he ought to follow. However, they may have some negative value by indicating lack of certain capacities. Certainly, they should not be used as the sole guide in deciding what occupation to follow!

41 *Nervous Diseases*

(The Brain, Spinal Cord, and Nerves)

What is the structure of the nervous system?

It is made up of the following:

a. The central nervous system, which includes the brain and spinal cord.

b. The peripheral nervous system, composed of those nerves which leave the spinal column and go to the various organs and structures in the body.

c. The autonomic (sympathetic) nervous system, composed of nerves which regulate the bowels, bladder, blood vessels, and functions of the body, such as sweating, heart rate, blood pressure, etc.

What are the cranial nerves?

These are twelve pairs of nerves extending from the brain through various openings in the skull, and supplying various structures in the face, head, and certain other organs.

What are the organs supplied by the various cranial nerves?

a. First nerves (olfactory) supply the nose and have to do with the sense of smell.

b. Second nerves (optic) are connected with the eyes and have to do with vision.

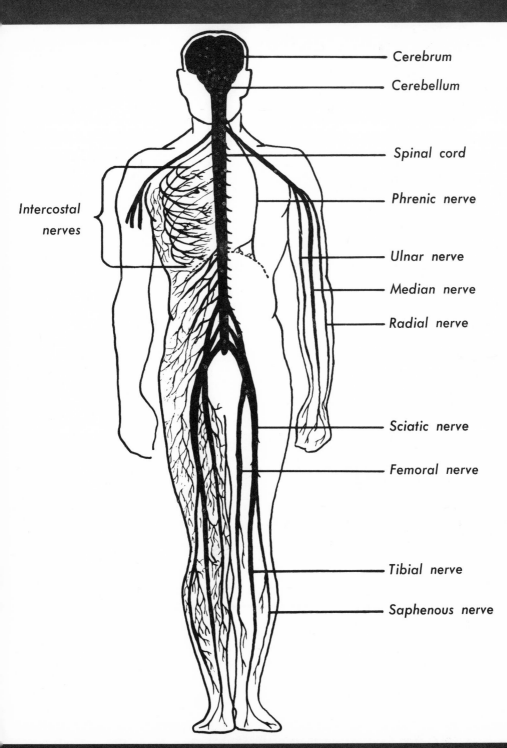

Cerebrum

Cerebellum

Spinal cord

Phrenic nerve

Intercostal
nerves

Ulnar nerve

Median nerve

Radial nerve

Sciatic nerve

Femoral nerve

Tibial nerve

Saphenous nerve

The Nervous System. This diagram shows the brain and its nerve attachments. Every part of the body is supplied by nerves, and all of these nerves connect with the brain. Some nerves carry impulses toward the brain: these are called afferent nerves. Other nerves carry impulses away from the brain: these are called efferent nerves. Nerve tissue shows very little tendency to regenerate, once it has been destroyed; thus we see relatively little recovery in people who have been paralyzed for more than several

c. Third, fourth, and sixth nerves control the movements of the eyeballs.

d. Fifth nerves (trigeminal) have to do with sensation in the face and control the muscles taking part in chewing.

e. Seventh (facial) nerves control the facial muscles.

f. Eighth nerves (acoustic and vestibular) have to do with hearing and the sense of balance.

g. Ninth (glossopharyngeal) nerves go to the throat and have to do with swallowing.

h. Tenth nerves (vagus) go to the heart, stomach, and the intestinal tract.

i. Eleventh (spinal accessory) nerves control certain muscles in the neck and shoulders.

j. Twelfth (hypoglossal) nerves control the tongue.

What are the spinal nerve roots?

The spinal cord has a pair of nerves, called roots, emerging at regular intervals from both sides of the cord. On each side, there is a posterior branch for sensation and an anterior for motor (muscular) control. These roots combine to form the peripheral nerves which are then distributed outside the spinal column to various organs and structures and muscles within the body. These nerves control all the muscles and glands and also control sensation all over the body.

What is the difference between a neurologist and a psychiatrist?

The neurologist studies and treats diseases which affect the structure of the nervous system. These are called organic diseases of the nervous system. The psychiatrist treats functional disorders of the brain, such as mental and emotional illness, neurosis, etc.

NEURITIS

What is neuritis?

Neuritis is a general term used to signify disease of the peripheral nerves. It may affect one nerve only, or it may be a diffuse process. Actually, neuritis is not a correct term, for very few of the diseases of nerves are due to actual inflammation. Modern terminology now classifies diseases of the nerves as neuropathy.

What are the causes of neuritis?

a. An accident causing direct injury to a single nerve.

b. Pressure upon a nerve due to a poorly healing fracture or to bone fragments or to a tumor which is growing and pressing upon the nerve.

c. Pressure upon a nerve as it exits from the spinal column, as in arthritis, or in the case of a herniated disc.

d. There may be many causes for neuritis of the diffuse type. This may be part of a deficiency disease such as one encounters with lack of vitamins (as in beriberi), etc. It may be seen with chronic alcoholism or in certain cases of advanced diabetes. Various toxic agents, such as lead, may affect the peripheral nerves and produce a neuritis. Finally, various generalized infections of the body may affect the peripheral nerves.

What is polyneuritis?

A term used to designate a condition in which many of the peripheral nerves are involved.

What are the symptoms of neuritis?

a. Tingling, described as pins and needles, and numbness in the hands and feet or in the region supplied by the nerve.

b. Muscular weakness and wasting of the muscles in the involved area.

c. Absent or reduced muscle reflexes in the area supplied by the involved nerves.

d. Loss of sensation in the affected part.

e. Pain, although this is not necessarily a constant finding in neuritis.

What is brachial neuritis?

It is a term applied to a painful nerve affliction of an arm. Brachial neuritis may be caused by a herniated disc in the vertebral column in the neck region or by a cervical rib, a condition in which there is an abnormal process on the lowest vertebra of the neck, causing pressure on some of the nerves going to the arm.

What is sciatica?

This is a term formerly used for a nerve disorder characterized by pain down the back of the thigh and leg. It is now known to be due, in most instances, to a herniated intervertebral disc in the lower back region. A true neuritis of the sciatic nerve may, however, occasionally occur and is most frequently encountered in advanced diabetes.

What is a herniated intervertebral disc?

It represents the displacement of the cartilage normally present between two adjacent vertebrae. This cartilage is called the intervertebral disc. Sometimes, as a result of arthritis, or as a result of a twisting injury to the spine, or in injuries of the spine occurring when one lifts a heavy object in a stooping position, this cartilage becomes displaced in such a way that it presses upon a nerve root which is exiting from the spinal column. This will cause severe pain along the course of that nerve. When the displacement occurs in the lower back (the lumbar region), the pain will radiate from the back to the buttocks and down the back of the thigh and leg. This can occur anywhere along the course of the spinal column and may cause pain and symptoms at the affected level. It is sometimes referred to as a slipped disc.

What is the treatment of herniated or slipped disc?

Early cases should be treated conservatively, with prolonged rest in bed. The patient should sleep on a mattress with a board under it. Heat to the area along the spinal column may prove helpful. Pain-relieving drugs, such as aspirin, may be used for purposes of obtaining relief. If prolonged rest does not help or if the pain recurs at frequent intervals and thus incapacitates the patient, surgery may become necessary. (See Chapter 42, on Neurosurgery.)

What is trigeminal neuralgia (tic doloureux)?

It is a disorder of the fifth cranial nerve, the trigeminal, which supplies the face. This is a very painful condition characterized by episodes of sudden excruciating pain in the face, coming in paroxysms and lasting for a short time. The attacks may be brought on by chewing, talking, exposure to cold, or by touching a sensitive point on the face or the mouth. These paroxysms of pain have a tendency to recur over a period of time varying from weeks to months. If the attacks become frequent and they do not subside readily, it may be necessary to inject the nerve in order to deaden it or it may become necessary to actually sever the nerve surgically. Cutting the affected portion of this nerve will cure the condition but will leave the patient with permanent numbness of that segment of the face supplied by the nerve. (See Chapter 42, on Neurosurgery.)

What is meant by "shingles"?

This disease is also called herpes zoster. It is an inflammation of one of the posterior roots of the spinal cord. It is characterized by severe, persistent burning pain and a skin eruption of small blisters along the course of the nerve.

What causes shingles?

It is believed to be caused by a virus, closely related to the one producing chickenpox.

What is the course of shingles?

The pain may be very severe and may last from a few to many weeks. In most cases, it subsides by itself.

What is the treatment for shingles?

There is no known specific treatment to cure this disease. Pain-relieving medications may be required. Many medications, x-ray treatments, and the injection of various substances have proved to be helpful in certain cases, but the great majority of patients must get well by themselves.

What is Bell's palsy (facial paralysis)?

It is an inflammation of the facial nerve resulting in paralysis of half of the face. The face and mouth sag on the affected side and the eye fails to close completely. It may occur at any age and affect either sex.

What is the cause of facial paralysis?

The cause is not known, but many people attribute it to having been exposed to a draft over a prolonged period of time.

What is the course of facial paralysis?

It usually lasts for two to three months and then has a tendency to clear up by itself.

Is complete recovery from facial paralysis usually the ultimate outcome?

Most cases make a near-complete recovery, but a small proportion of people are left with some permanent weakness of the involved side of the face.

What is the treatment for facial paralysis?

Since the eye fails to close completely, it should be protected by having the patient wear glasses that enclose the entire eye or by placing a small shield to the side of the face. Electrical stimulation with electric machines is often applied to the weak facial muscles, but the value of this form of treatment has not been proved conclusively. The general health of the patient should be maintained and the patient should have an adequate diet and vitamin intake. There is no known specific treatment which will bring about a more rapid cure.

CEREBRAL PALSY

What is cerebral palsy?

This is not a single disease but a group of neurological disorders affecting children and beginning at birth. Children with cerebral palsy have difficulty in walking and may have many involuntary movements of the limbs and muscles of the face. It often affects speech and makes it blurred and difficult to understand. There may be no mental impairment, or mental impairment may, in some cases, be severe. The muscular condition is characterized by a stiffness or spasticity of the limbs, resulting in awkward or stiff-legged gait.

What causes cerebral palsy?

It is thought that a difficult labor, an excessively prolonged labor, or lack of oxygen to the unborn infant during labor may be the cause of certain cases. Some cases are due to actual injury to the brain during delivery. Others are due to a disorder within the germ cells which is passed on to the infant; that is, in some there is a hereditary basis. Some cases are thought to be the result of illness in the mother during the first twelve weeks of pregnancy. Also, certain cases are thought to be due to cysts of the brain with which the child is born.

Is there any effective treatment for cerebral palsy?

Yes. Children with cerebral palsy can be greatly benefited by persistent and prolonged education and other physical measures aimed toward rehabilitation and better control of muscles.

Should children with cerebral palsy be sent to special schools, if possible?

Yes. The rehabilitation methods being used today are a striking advance over former years. Excellent results are now being obtained by special educators in this particular field of rehabilitation.

Does cerebral palsy get worse as the child grows older, and does it result in premature death?

No. The children tend to improve as they reach adulthood, and many of these people lead normal, healthy lives.

HYDROCEPHALUS

What is hydrocephalus?

This is sometimes called "water on the brain." It is due to the excessive accumulation of cerebrospinal fluid within the ventricles of the brain. This leads to enlargement of the infant's head as the child grows.

What is the actual physical cause of hydrocephalus?

An obstruction to the flow of spinal fluid from the brain down to the spinal canal.

What happens to the brain in a child with hydrocephalus?

There is progressive deterioration or loss of brain substance from the pressure of the accumulated fluid, and this results in progressive deterioration in brain function.

Can a tumor within the brain or an inflammation of the brain due to infection cause hydrocephalus?

Yes, in certain cases.

Can hydrocephalus be helped?

New surgical approaches to this disease are producing an occasional good result. (See Chapter 42, on Neurosurgery.)

BRAIN TUMORS

Are brain tumors common?

Yes. The brain is one of the most frequent sites for tumor formation.

What symptoms do brain tumors cause?

a. Persistent and recurring headaches.
b. Progressive weakness of an arm or leg or perhaps more than one limb at a time.
c. Disturbances in sensation, such as numbness.
d. Impairment of vision, such as double vision or loss of sight in one eye.
e. Dizziness or vertigo.
f. Convulsions.
g. Sudden episodes of headache and vomiting.

Are most headaches indicative of brain tumor?

Absolutely not. Headaches alone, unaccompanied by other of the symptoms listed above, are rarely caused by brain tumors.

How are brain tumors diagnosed?

The neurologist and the neurosurgeon have many competent methods of investigating brain tumors. These will include examination of the eye grounds, thorough neurological investigation of the function of all of the nerves of the body, special x-rays employing the injection of air or opaque liquids to demonstrate brain or blood vessel outlines, and the employment of electroencephalography.

Are brain tumors ever curable?

Yes, some forms are. (See Chapter 42, on Neurosurgery.)

ENCEPHALITIS

What is encephalitis?

An acute inflammation of the brain.

What are some of the symptoms of encephalitis?

Headache, fever, vomiting, paralysis, delirium, convulsions, stupor, and, in some cases, coma.

What causes encephalitis?

Any one of a number of viruses. It may also occur as a complication of measles, whooping cough, or mumps. Infrequently, it may occur with severe infections, such as pneumonia and typhoid fever, or as a toxic reaction accompanying any disease with prolonged high fever.

Is encephalitis ever seen in an epidemic form?

Yes, most often during war periods and in war camps. It is also seen in localized areas involving a town or city.

What is the treatment of encephalitis?

Unfortunately, there is no specific treatment.

What is the outcome of encephalitis?

The majority of patients will recover completely. However, when the disease exists in epidemic form, there may be a considerable initial mortality. There may also be partial recovery in some patients who will be left with serious mental deficiencies.

885

Is encephalitis sometimes called "sleeping sickness"?

Yes.

Does encephalitis ever lead to the development of symptoms years after the acute attack?

Yes. Certain people who have recovered from encephalitis may develop tremors, palsies, and various other disorders later on.

MENINGITIS

What is meningitis?

An infection of the coverings of the brain and spinal cord.

What are the symptoms of meningitis?

The rather abrupt onset of fever, severe headache, stiff neck, and, often, coma. On tapping the spine, inflammation may be discovered in the spinal fluid, and examination of the spinal fluid under the microscope will reveal inflammatory cells or even the germ which has caused the meningitis.

What are the various causes of meningitis?

Some are caused by infection with pus-forming bacteria, others may be due to an infection spreading from the middle ear or the sinuses. Other types of acute meningitis are caused by viruses. There are still other types of meningitis occurring with tuberculosis and syphilis.

How is the diagnosis of meningitis made definitely?

By tapping the spine and analyzing the spinal fluid.

What is the treatment for meningitis?

This would depend completely upon the causative agent. Those types caused by the pus-forming bacteria can be successfully treated with the antibiotics or with the sulfa drugs. Most of the types caused by viruses must be treated symptomatically.

Special treatment is now available for meningitis caused by tuberculosis or syphilis.

Can meningitis be cured?

Yes. The great majority can now be cured by the newer drugs that are available.

SYPHILIS OF THE NERVOUS SYSTEM

How does syphilis affect the nervous system?

In former years, syphilis was a common cause of diseases of the nervous system. Modern treatment of syphilis has now been so successful that this is a rare disease today. One variety, still seen occasionally, is syphilitic meningitis.

What is paresis (general paralysis)?

This was a disease encounted much more frequently years ago, when syphilis involved the brain itself. It resulted chiefly in a mental disorder.

What is locomotor ataxia (tabes)?

This is a disease in which syphilis mainly affects the spinal cord and leads to a staggering gait.

Can syphilis of the nervous system be treated effectively today?

Yes. The antibiotics are very effective in treating this disease if it is diagnosed during its earlier stages.

CEREBROVASCULAR ACCIDENTS
("Strokes")

What are cerebrovascular accidents?

These are commonly called a stroke or apoplexy. These conditions are the result of a more or less abrupt interruption of the blood supply to some area of the brain.

How do strokes or apoplexy take place?

Usually, in one of three ways:

a. By a cerebral thrombosis or the clotting of a blood vessel in the brain.

b. By cerebral hemorrhage, which means the rupture of one of the blood vessels to the brain.

c. By cerebral embolism, or a blood clot from elsewhere in the body being distributed to a blood vessel in the brain, thus blocking the vessel.

What is cerebral thrombosis?

A form of stroke in which an artery which is the seat of arterio-sclerosis has undergone thickening and hardening of its wall and the interior of the vessel, and has thereby become reduced so that blood fails to flow through it. The area of brain normally supplied by that blood vessel will no longer receive blood, and this affected area will become degenerated and die. The function normally provided by that brain area is lost, and certain symptoms and signs may appear. Loss of speech and partial paralysis of one or more limbs are frequently seen following cerebral thrombosis. Paralysis of one-half of the body (hemiplegia) may occur in some cases.

What causes cerebral hemorrhage?

In another variety of stroke, an area of the brain is the seat of hemorrhage. This occurs when a blood vessel, small or large, ruptures. This occurs most frequently in people with high blood pressure or in a disease wherein bleeding takes place. When a large blood vessel is involved, the patient may die rather quickly. If the blood vessel is small, only a small area of brain may be damaged and the patient may make a recovery. The functions normally provided by that area of the brain will cease and the patient may develop symptoms similar to those caused by cerebral thrombosis.

Does cerebral hemorrhage ever occur in young people?

Once in a very great while, when there has been an abnormality in the formation of a blood vessel. In these instances, a blood vessel may rupture as a result of a defect in its wall.

What is cerebral embolism?

A condition in which a blood vessel is blocked by a clot or other fragment traveling to the brain from some distant site. This may arise from phlebitis (inflammation of a vein) which has developed in some other part of the body or, more frequently, from a clot which has formed on the wall of a heart which has been affected by rheumatic fever or a coronary occlusion.

What are some of the common symptoms of a stroke?

a. Loss of consciousness.
b. Weakness and paralysis of one side of the body.
c. The exact symptom will depend upon the area of the brain which has been affected by the stroke.

What is the course of the patient who has had a stroke?

This will depend upon how large a blood vessel has been affected and how much brain tissue has been damaged. Death may result quickly or in a few days if the blood vessel is large and the area of brain damage is extensive. Many strokes are much less severe, probably the majority, and after a variable period of time the patient gradually recovers. Such patients will usually retain some degree of weakness, stiffness, and partial paralysis in the involved arm or leg.

Some strokes are mild, so that there is no loss of consciousness, and the patient may merely have weakness in one limb for a short period of time, perhaps for only a few hours. This occurs in some cases of hypertension (high blood pressure) and is usually attributed to spasm of an artery in the brain. It is seen most often in older people and is termed a minor stroke.

How can one tell if a patient who has had a stroke will recover?

The outlook for a patient who has had a stroke improves with the passage of time. Those who survive the first few days have a much better chance to get well. Also, when the patient has not lost consciousness, it is a favorable prognostic sign.

Do people who have recovered from a stroke regain normal mental states?

Yes, very often. Those who recover are usually mentally alert and normal. Even those who have lost the ability to speak, retain the ability to understand things fully.

Can a patient who has lost the power of speech as the result of a stroke be retrained to speak?

Excellent new work in speech rehabilitation has been developed within recent years. Many of these people, who are not too far along in years, can be trained to speak again.

Will the paralysis that results from a stroke tend to diminish as one recovers from the condition?

Yes. Also, in this type of case, modern methods of rehabilitation enable people who have had strokes to make excellent recoveries.

EPILEPSY

What is epilepsy?

A disorder characterized by convulsions, or seizures, or spells, in which there is temporary loss of consciousness or memory. Since there are many causes for these seizures, the epilepsy may only be a symptom. Neurologists, therefore, prefer to use the term "convulsive state," rather than epilepsy.

Are there different types of epileptic seizures?

Yes, there is the so-called *grand mal*, which is a generalized convulsion. There is also the *petit mal*, meaning a small attack, in which the patient has a brief lapse of contact with his surroundings, after which he will resume where he left off.

What are the common symptoms of the major epileptic convulsions?

a. Loss of consciousness.
b. Shaking convulsions, in which the arms and legs undergo strong repetitive to and fro movements for a short period of time.
c. Biting of the tongue and frothing at the mouth.
d. The patient may soil or wet himself.

What are the causes of epilepsy?

a. It may be caused by any condition or disease affecting the brain, such as a brain tumor or scars secondary to a brain injury or infection.

b. It may be caused by a birth injury.

c. There may be hereditary epilepsy.

d. There are a great number of patients with epilepsy in whom the cause is unknown. Certain cases of epilepsy are thought to be psychological in origin.

What is the usual age at which epilepsy has its onset?

It begins most often at puberty, but may appear even in earlier childhood.

Does epilepsy affect both sexes equally?

Yes.

Are people with epilepsy mentally retarded or below average in mentality?

Not necessarily. Many of them are normal or even above average in intelligence.

Can epilepsy ever be cured?

Yes, if the cause can be determined and removed. (See Chapter 42, on Neurosurgery.)

Can epilepsy be controlled?

Yes. The great majority of cases can be controlled so that the seizures are reduced to a minimum. There are excellent medications on the market which tend to reduce or eliminate the convulsions.

Is epilepsy of psychological origin ever curable?

Yes, in certain instances, by prolonged psychotherapy.

What is the first-aid treatment for a patient who is having a convulsion?

Guard him from injury. If he is on the floor, let him remain there. Put a pillow under his head. Do *not* attempt to force anything between his teeth.

How frequently is epilepsy encountered?

Statistics tend to show that about 1 per cent of all people have epilepsy.

Is epilepsy inherited?

From 10 to 25 per cent of patients will give a history of epilepsy in some other member of the family. However, it is important to note that there is only a one in ten chance that a child in a family in which there is epilepsy, will develop the condition. If one parent has epilepsy, the chance of a child developing epilepsy is only one in forty.

Is epilepsy a bar to marriage?

No.

Should an epileptic have children?

If there is an evident cause for the epilepsy, heredity will play no part and the patient can have children without any hesitation. If there is a family history of epilepsy on one side only, the chances of having epileptic children are very slight. Where there is a positive family history on both sides, serious consideration should be given to not having children.

Does a child who has a convulsion associated with high fever or some childhood disease have epilepsy?

No. Usually, this is a different kind of condition, having no association with true epilepsy. Sometimes, however, convulsions during fever in early childhood are followed by epilepsy later on.

Should epileptics be permitted to live a normal life and to engage in a gainful occupation?

Yes. They can be taught how to keep medicated so that their chances of getting a seizure are minimal. They should follow such occupations as will not be dangerous should a seizure occur.

What are the precautions that an epileptic should take?

a. Do not drive an automobile unless one is sure that the attacks are well controlled with medication.

b. Never drink alcohol.

c. Do not swim alone.

d. Limit total fluid intake to approximately three or four glasses per day.

e. Always take medications at regular intervals, follow medical instructions carefully, and *never* stop medication without consulting your doctor.

f. Avoid unnecessary stress and emotional strain.

g. Do not permit the supply of medication to fall so low that one may run out of it.

FAINTING

What is fainting?

Fainting, or syncope, is a brief, temporary loss of consciousness resulting from a transient reduction in the circulation of blood to the brain.

What are some of the causes of fainting?

a. Emotional upset.

b. Too sudden a fall in blood sugar (hypoglycemia).

c. An overdose of insulin in a diabetic patient.

d. Certain heart conditions.

e. Extreme pain.

Do patients ever die in a faint?

This is extremely rare, as most patients who faint will regain consciousness by themselves.

What should be done for a patient who has fainted?

See that he lies flat and that his head is at a level with or below the level of the rest of his body. Loosen the patient's collar so that he can breathe easily.

893

C O M A

What is coma?

It is a state of unconsciousness from which the patient cannot be aroused.

What are some of the more common causes of coma?

There are many:

a. A toxic agent, such as excessive alcohol or excessive consumption of sleeping pills.

b. Severe brain injury, such as in concussion or fractured skull.

c. Severe infection, such as meningitis or encephalitis.

d. A brain tumor or a stroke due to a cerebral hemorrhage or thrombosis.

e. A complication of diabetes due to an excessively high blood sugar, with accompanying acidosis.

f. Uremia, with failure of kidney function.

g. Hysteria, secondary to severe emotional upset.

What is the treatment of coma?

To ascertain the cause and to treat it. Hence, diagnosis is the most important initial step. Patients who are in coma should be hospitalized immediately so that the various tests can be instituted which will determine the cause.

H E A D A C H E

What is the significance of headache?

Headaches are among the most common of symptoms and frequently constitute the most difficult problem confronting both physician and patient. Headache is a symptom, not a disease. As such, headache may occur from a wide variety of disorders. It may be associated with disease involving some of the structures about the head, such as the eyes, the nose, the sinuses, or the ears. It may be due to disease of structures within the head involving the brain. Most often, however, it is the result of emotional disturbance. Another frequent cause of headache is a general disturbance within the body, such as a systemic disease with fever.

Are headaches ever caused by allergies?

Yes.

Is headache ever caused by excessive fatigue or tension?

Yes.

Should a patient with frequent headaches consult his physician?

Yes.

What is migraine?

This is a very common condition characterized by recurring paroxysmal headache, occurring in bouts, often affecting one side of the head. Between attacks, the patient feels perfectly well.

What is the cause of migraine?

The cause is unknown, but it frequently affects several members of a family.

Is emotional tension ever a cause of migraine?

Yes.

Can migraine ever be cured?

Yes, if one is able to determine its cause and to treat it along those lines.

Will a competent neurologist be able to distinguish between a headache caused by a serious nerve or brain disease and one which is caused by a trivial condition or an emotional upset?

Yes. The neurologist has many methods for distinguishing the various causes of headache.

Does headache ever respond to psychotherapy?

Inasmuch as the great majority of headaches are caused by emotional upset, prolonged psychotherapy often leads to their cure.

VERTIGO

What is vertigo?

It is a symptom in which there is a sense of rotation of one's surroundings or a sense of loss of balance in space so that one is unable to maintain his equilibrium.

What is the importance of vertigo?

It indicates a disturbance of the vestibular apparatus. This is the organ of equilibrium and it includes its nerve connections with the brain. Hence, disease at any point in this system may cause vertigo. Included in this are diseases of the inner ear, neuritis, and tumors of the eighth cranial nerve, diseases within the brain, etc.

MENIÈRE'S DISEASE

What is Menière's disease?

An illness characterized by sudden paroxysms of vertigo, nausea, and vomiting, in which the patient lies down and is unable to move because of loss of equilibrium. Usually, the paroxysm is of short duration, lasting anywhere from minutes to hours. It subsides gradually, and the patient is then well for long intervals. During the acute disturbance there may be noises in one ear, such as buzzing, hissing, or whistling. After a number of such attacks there may be decreased hearing in that ear. The cause for this disease is not definitely known but has been attributed to increased fluid or edema in the inner ear.

What is the treatment for Menière's disease?

In the acute phase, there must be complete rest. Sedatives and other medication may be helpful. Fluid intake should be limited and salt eliminated from the diet. Medicines are given to reduce the water content of the body.

MUSCULAR DYSTROPHY

What is muscular dystrophy?

An inherited muscular disorder usually affecting several members of one family. It often begins in childhood and is evidenced by various muscles becoming weak, with progressive weakening of the hips, the thighs, back muscles, shoulders, and arms. Such patients have trouble in walking, in rising from the prone position, and in elevating their arms. Ultimately, the muscles will waste away, although there may be a temporary phase of the disease in which some muscles appear enlarged.

What is the outlook for muscular dystrophy?

The condition is likely to progress slowly and become worse over a period of years. Although the condition may seem to become arrested for a time, there is ultimate progression to a fatal outcome.

MULTIPLE SCLEROSIS
(*Disseminated Sclerosis*)

What is multiple sclerosis?

A disease of the central nervous system resulting in what is called demyelination, or loss of the myelin sheaths which cover the nerve fibers. This occurs usually in small patches and is characterized clinically by the rapid development of symptoms which prevail for a varying period of time and then recede. A period of freedom from symptoms is called a remission. Later, additional episodes occur which also tend to remit. The average case displays a series of intermittent and remittent illnesses affecting various parts of the nervous system. In most people the disorder is progressive, although the rate of progress varies markedly in different cases. Common symptoms are:

a. Temporary loss of vision in one or the other eye.

b. Temporary weakness of limbs, awkwardness, and clumsiness of movement (termed ataxia).

897

c. Stiffness of the limbs (spasticity).

d. Bladder trouble resulting in loss of urine or difficulty in voiding, etc.

What is the cause of multiple sclerosis?

The cause is unknown.

What is the outlook for a patient with multiple sclerosis?

This is a progressive disease which ultimately leaves the patient bedridden. It may take many years to reach such a state and some fortunate people may live out an almost normal life span without becoming too greatly incapacitated.

Is there any effective treatment for multiple sclerosis?

At this time there is no specific cure. Many forms of treatment have been helpful, but none is consistently successful. Many of the symptoms can be alleviated, and it must be remembered that the natural history of this disease includes long periods of spontaneous improvement.

PARKINSONISM
(Shaking Palsy)

What is Parkinsonism?

A disease of the brain characterized by muscular rigidity and tremor. The rigidity is of a particular kind which slows up all movements and produces an expressionless face. The tremor, or shaking, is rhythmic, slow, and is present even when the patient is resting. It may affect one or both sides of the body. This disorder affects middle-aged and elderly people, and is generally progressive, though often very slowly so. Ultimately, patients tend to become helpless. The condition is also known as paralysis agitans, although actual paralysis does not occur.

What is the cause of Parkinsonism?

Most varieties are due to hardening of the cerebral arteries or are the result of brain damage caused by a previous illness such as encephalitis. Others are caused by degeneration of certain parts of the brain.

Is there any effective medical treatment for Parkinsonism?

Yes. A number of medications are available which are very helpful. Also, psychotherapy is of benefit to some patients and helps to keep them active physically and socially by helping them adjust to and accept their illness.

Can surgery ever be helpful in Parkinsonism?

Yes. (See Chapter 42, on Neurosurgery.)

FRACTURED SKULL

How serious is a skull fracture?

Skull fractures are serious, but by far the majority of cases will eventually get well. If there is no associated brain injury or depression of the bones with pressure upon the brain, recovery is almost always the outcome. Fortunately, most skull fractures are linear breaks without displacement, and these are not too serious. What is important in any head injury is what happens to the brain. Thus, head injury may be serious without a skull fracture, whereas a head injury with a long skull fracture may be relatively unimportant.

What is the outlook for skull fracture?

Very good, unless complicated by depression of a fracture fragment, a break in the skin, laceration of brain substance, or hemorrhage within the brain.

What is the management for skull fracture?

If there is no serious underlying brain damage, treatment should be symptomatic and should include bed rest for a few days and sedatives and analgesics to relieve head pain. If there is depression of a fracture fragment pressing upon the brain, or if there is brain hemorrhage, these complications must be treated surgically. (See Chapter 42, on Neurosurgery.)

CEREBRAL CONCUSSION

What is cerebral concussion?

It is a head injury accompanied by a short period of unconsciousness. It is often followed by headaches and dizzy feelings for some period of time. Concussion is usually not disabling, though often it is associated with moderate emotional disturbance, anxiety, and worry.

What is the outlook for cerebral concussion?

Ultimate recovery almost invariably takes place. However, some patients tend to have recurring headache or dizziness at varying intervals for an indeterminate period, occasionally for many months. Emotional disturbance is often present and tends to increase and prolong the symptoms. Older patients and emotionally unstable people are more apt to have prolonged symptoms.

Does cerebral concussion affect the mind?

No.

Is cerebral concussion likely to cause serious trouble at a later date?

The great majority make a complete recovery. There are, however, a small number of people who, as a result of a head injury, develop a blood clot around the brain. This is known as a subdural hematoma. It evidences itself many weeks or months later by progressive symptoms which will require neurosurgery for removal of the blood clot. Therefore, it is wise for people who have had even minor head injuries to receive periodic physical examinations by a neurologist as long as any symptoms persist.

What is the post-concussion syndrome or the post-traumatic state?

It is a group of symptoms which often follows cerebral concussion, and includes headache and dizziness. There may also be excessive fatigue and lack of energy, a feeling of pressure on the head, and inability to carry on sustained work. Emotional factors are also encountered, with worry and depression being seen quite often.

What is the treatment of the post-concussion syndrome?

Psychotherapy is most important. It must be sustained, prolonged, persistent, and frequent. Suitable employment within the tolerance of the patient and with due recognition and assessment of his disability is important.

Are the headaches and dizziness following concussion ever permanent?

No. Sooner or later, these symptoms will subside.

LUMBAR PUNCTURE
(Spinal Tap)

What is a lumbar puncture, and why is it performed?

It is a procedure or test which yields a sample of the cerebrospinal fluid. This fluid bathes the brain and the central nervous system. By this test, it is possible to measure directly the intracranial pressure and thereby detect any increase in pressure, such as occurs with tumors of the brain. The constituents of this fluid are altered in different ways by different diseases of the central nervous system. This test is often very necessary and yields information of the greatest importance to the doctor in diagnosing and managing the patient's illness. Thus, with infections of the nervous system, the examinaion of the cerebrospinal fluid helps to prove the presence of infection and to determine the nature of the infecting organism. At times, there is reluctance and resistance on the part of the patient or family to this procedure because of the mistaken idea that the test is dangerous or disabling. This is not true. The procedure is quite simple and harmless.

PNEUMOENCEPHALOGRAPHY

What is pneumoencephalography?

This is a special form of x-ray of the brain and contents of the skull. In this procedure, air is injected into the space around the brain and spinal cord by way of a spinal puncture. The air finds its way into the ventricles (normal cavities) of the brain, and since it is transparent to the x-rays it may disclose any distortion or enlargement of these cavities. Encephalography often reveals the presence and location of a brain tumor.

901

Is there any risk involved in pneumoencephalography?

Yes. There is some risk but it is small, and when carried out in a well-equipped hospital there are few complications. Any risk must be balanced against the risk of not knowing fully the patient's exact illness. In order to treat brain conditions accurately, neurologists and neurosurgeons must have every bit of exact information that it is possible to ascertain.

VENTRICULOGRAPHY

What is ventriculography?

This is an x-ray test in which air is injected directly into the ventricles of the brain through a surgical opening made in the skull. This

Electroencephalograph Machine and Patient. Here the electrodes are being placed upon the scalp. An electroencephalogram records the brain waves, and by noting abnormalities in these waves, diagnosis of brain disease can often be made.

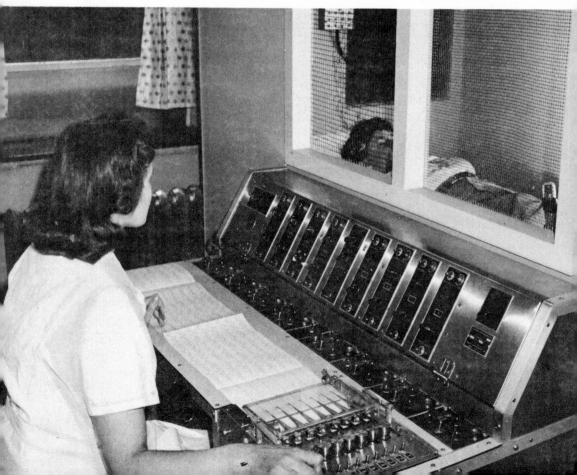

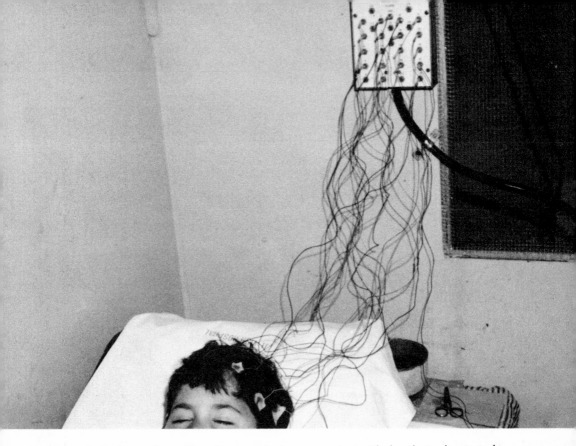

Electroencephalography. This photograph shows a patient with the electrodes pasted at various sites on the scalp. Electroencephalography is a painless procedure and causes little or no discomfort.

procedure is applicable when there are signs of increased pressure within the brain and when it is inadvisable to inject air through the spinal route.

ELECTROENCEPHALOGRAPHY

What is electroencephalography?

This is a procedure which records the minute quantity of electrical activity normally going on in the brain and which reflects brain activity. A system of considerable magnification makes this activity visible on a strip of paper, in the form of waves. Hence, these are called the "brain waves." The normal pattern is quite characteristic and is often modified by disease of the brain. Thus, epilepsy causes typical changes in the brain waves. Tumors, strokes, and injuries may alter the pattern in a special way. For convenience, the procedure is referred to by the abbreviation E.E.G.

Is electroencephalography a helpful and accurate diagnostic aid in brain disease?

Yes, but it should not be used as the sole test. When used along with other diagnostic tests, it is most valuable.

Brain Wave Tracings. These electroencephalographic tracings show essentially normal brain waves. Although normal brain wave tracings will not exclude completely the possibility of brain disease, they are helpful diagnostic aids.

904

42 *Neurosurgery*

(Brain, Spinal Cord, and Nerve Surgery)

What is the scope of neurosurgery?

Neurosurgery is that branch of medicine dealing with the surgical treatment of diseases of the nervous system, including the brain, spinal cord, and peripheral nerves. Injuries, infections, tumors, various congenital abnormalities, ruptured discs, certain painful states, and intracranial hemorrhage are among the conditions which can be helped by the neurosurgeon.

Generally speaking, how does the nervous system function?

The nervous system is composed of nerve cells and supporting tissue centered in the brain and spinal cord, with widespread extensions all through the body. Its function is the transmission and coordination of stimuli and their integration into the phenomena which make up mental activity. Impulses conveying sensory impressions, such as touch, taste, hearing, sight, and smell, are carried to the brain along pathways called afferent nerves. Glandular secretion and muscular activity, on the other hand, are achieved by impulses which originate in the central nervous system and travel in an outward direction along pathways called efferent nerves.

The orderliness which characterizes normal human activity is rendered possible only because of the high degree of organization of the nervous system. This fact becomes apparent when a part of this elaborate system is disturbed by a disease process.

The nervous system is divided anatomically into two components, a central and a peripheral. The brain and spinal cord make up the central portion; the peripheral part is composed of all the nerves which establish communication with the rest of the body. The peripheral component consists of twelve pairs of cranial nerves which arise from the brain and leave through openings in the bones of the skull, thirty-one pairs of spinal nerves which emerge through openings in the vertebral column, and a complex network of nerves called the autonomic or sympathetic system. The function of the autonomic system is to transmit nervous impulses to the intestinal tract, bladder, heart, glands, and blood vessels.

What is the appearance of the brain?

The brain is a soft, grayish-white structure, hemispheral in shape, with innumerable folds. It is nourished by many blood vessels which permeate its substance. It is continuous with the spinal cord, which emerges through an opening in the base of the skull.

Both the brain and spinal cord are covered by membranes (the dura, arachnoid and pia) and by a liquid called cerebrospinal fluid. Within the brain itself are a number of communicating cavities also containing cerebrospinal fluid.

How does one gain surgical access to the brain?

The operation for exposing the brain is called a craniotomy. As a general rule, craniotomy is performed under general anesthesia, though at times local anesthesia is preferable. In preparation for surgery, the entire head is shaved and the scalp cleansed thoroughly with soap and water. A skin antiseptic is then applied, and all but the area to be operated upon is covered with sterile drapes. The scalp is incised, usually in a semicircular manner, and a number of holes are drilled in the underlying skull. The holes are connected by means of a wire saw, thereby freeing a block of bone which is detached from the remainder of the skull. Directly underneath the bone are the membranes overlying the brain. These are incised, thus exposing the brain.

Progress in surgical technique has made it possible to gain access to almost any part of the brain with reasonable safety!

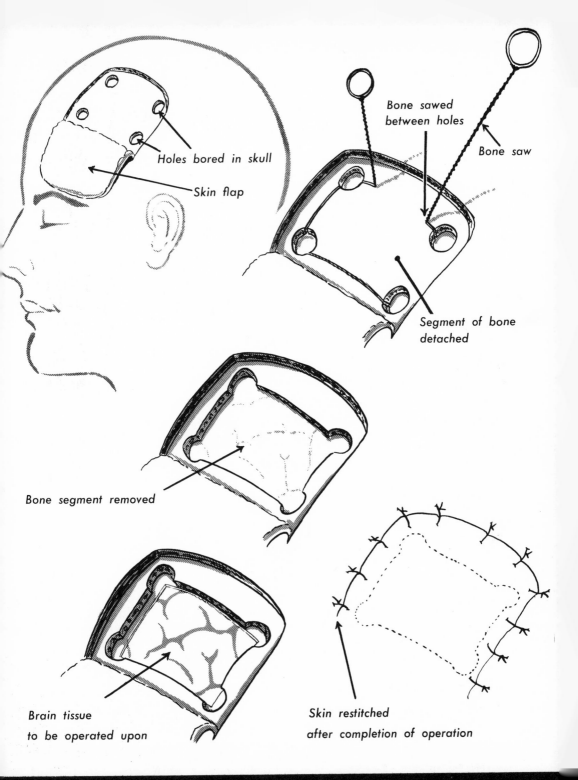

Holes bored in skull

Skin flap

Bone sawed between holes

Bone saw

Segment of bone detached

Bone segment removed

Brain tissue to be operated upon

Skin restitched after completion of operation

Craniotomy. Surgical approach for a brain operation. Brain surgery has advanced so remarkably within the last twenty to thirty years that it is not much more dangerous than surgery upon any other region of the body. Incisions for brain operations are

What is the appearance and function of the spinal cord?

The spinal cord is an elongated, cylindrically shaped structure which measures approximately eighteen inches in length and occupies the canal within the vertebral column. It consists of bundles of nerves and its function is to act primarily as a conducting mechanism. Sensory impulses travel toward the brain, while impulses concerned with muscular contraction and movement descend in the opposite direction. Connections with various organs and structures are established by means of spinal nerves which are attached to the cord throughout its length.

How is the spinal cord exposed?

An incision is made in the center of the back, and the muscles overlying the spinal column are spread apart. Parts of the arches of the exposed vertebrae are then removed, thereby bringing into view the spinal cord enclosed within its membranes. This operation is known as a laminectomy.

SKULL AND BRAIN INJURIES
(Lacerations, Concussion, Fracture)

Are all head injuries serious?

No, on the contrary, head injuries vary in seriousness from the relatively minor laceration of the scalp to the severe bruising of the brain associated with profound unconsciousness. Fortunately, the skull affords considerable protection to the underlying brain substance. Many head injuries damage only the relatively unimportant superficial tissues. Those of a more severe nature may fracture the skull and cause serious brain damage, such as a laceration or contusion.

Is a laceration of the scalp serious?

Scalp lacerations frequently look more serious than they really are, because of their great tendency to bleed. The bleeding usually stops by itself or after pressure has been applied. Surgical repair of the wound is necessary in cases of extensive laceration. The hair around the wound is shaved and the laceration cleansed before it is sutured.

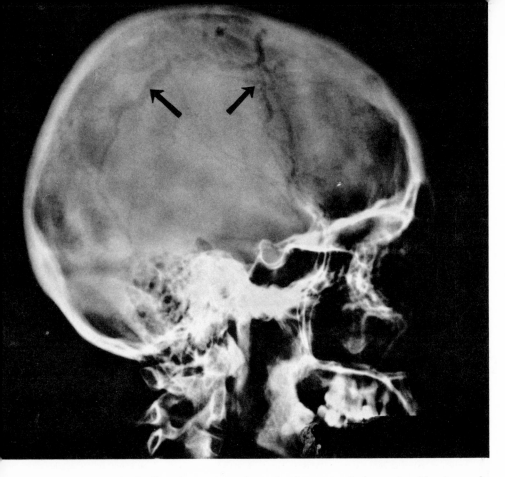

X-ray of Normal Skull. The arrows show the location of the major blood vessels which supply the brain. Skull x-rays can tell the presence of bone deformities, fractures, and in some instances tumors.

Careful inspection of the wound is necessary to be certain that the injury has not involved the skull or underlying brain.

What is the significance of loss of consciousness following a head injury?

It signifies that an injury to the intracranial contents has taken place! X-rays should always be taken in such cases because of the possibility of a skull fracture. Patients who have lost consciousness, if only for a few seconds, should be observed carefully for a day or two for evidence of hemorrhage within the skull.

What is meant by a concussion?

Concussion is a term applied to a head injury that has resulted in loss of consciousness for a brief period.

What is the treatment for a concussion?

No specific treatment is required in uncomplicated cases, as spontaneous recovery is the rule. The patient should, however, be watched for the development of increasing drowsiness and weakness of the limbs on one side of the body. Such symptoms are usually caused by bleeding within the skull.

Is a fractured skull a serious injury?

Yes. Skull fractures result from a severe blow or fall upon the head. However, it must be emphasized that it is not the extent of the fracture that determines the seriousness of the injury, but the amount of damage to the underlying brain. In other words, a small fracture accompanied by widespread brain damage may be much more dangerous than an extensive skull fracture that has caused little brain damage.

Is the patient's state of consciousness an important factor in regard to the severity of the injury as well as the ultimate outcome?

Yes. The depth and duration of coma or stupor vary in proportion to the severity of the injury.

What is the proper first-aid treatment for a head injury with loss of consciousness?

a. Place the patient on his side or in a semi-prone position.

b. Hemorrhage from a scalp wound should be controlled by pressure with a sterile dressing or clean handkerchief.

c. Transport the patient on a stretcher; avoid bending his head or trunk.

Is there any specific treatment for injury to the brain?

No. There is no specific treatment for brain injuries as such. Fortunately, most patients recover spontaneously.

Is it necessary to operate on all cases of head injury?

No.

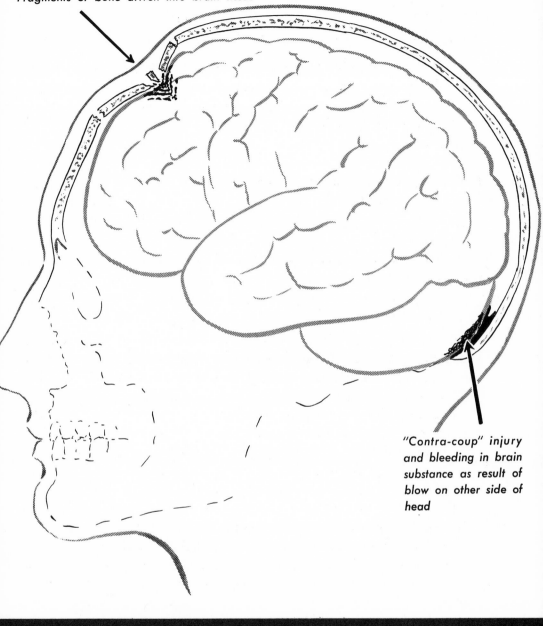

Fragments of bone driven into brain tissue

"Contra-coup" injury and bleeding in brain substance as result of blow on other side of head

Depressed Skull Fracture. This diagram shows a depressed skull fracture with some of the bone fragments being driven in toward the brain substance. This is a serious condition demanding surgery to relieve the pressure which such bone fragments might create upon the brain. Often a severe blow on one side of the skull will produce a hemorrhage or laceration of brain substance on the opposite side of the skull. Such a condition is called a "contre coup" injury, as shown in the above diagram.

What are the indications for surgery?

a. An open wound (i.e., compound fracture).

b. The presence of indriven or depressed fragments of bone which may irritate the brain (depressed skull fracture).

c. Intracranial hemorrhage developing as a complication.

d. A persistent leak of cerebrospinal fluid through the nose.

Is the occurrence of bleeding within the skull following a head injury a serious complication?

Yes.

How does intracranial hemorrhage following injury manifest itself, and what can be done about it?

Evidence of hemorrhage within the skull may appear within a matter of hours after an injury or may be delayed for weeks, or even months. Seemingly slight injuries may be followed by intracranial bleeding; thus, a careful lookout for this complication must be maintained. Intracranial bleeding occurring soon after an accident constitutes a surgical emergency. It is manifested by increasing drowsiness and weakness of the limbs on one side of the body. Prompt recognition of the condition and operation to stop the bleeding and remove the blood clots are imperative to avoid a fatal outcome. Even the suspicion of hemorrhage is sufficient to warrant an immediate exploratory operation. This is a relatively minor operative procedure, performed under local novocaine anesthesia. A small incision is made in the scalp in front of and above the ear and a hole is drilled in the skull. Should the exploration fail to disclose the presence of a hemorrhage, no harm will have been done. On the other hand, failure to operate when a clot is present will cost the patient his life!

The symptoms of hemorrhage which appear at a late stage, weeks or months after an injury, consist of headache, drowsiness, and mental confusion. This type of bleeding presents a much less urgent problem, although treatment is similar to that for the more acute variety. Blood clots may be evacuated through a small opening in the skull, although at times a more extensive surgical procedure is necessary.

Does intracranial bleeding ever occur during early life?

Yes. Intracranial hemorrhage (subdural hematoma, or clot over-lying the brain) resulting from injury is sometimes encountered during infancy. The trauma may have occurred inadvertently at the time the baby was born. Early diagnosis and surgical treatment are essential to prevent permanent brain damage.

Is physical or mental disability a common sequel of head injury?

Considering the frequency with which head injuries occur, the incidence of serious after-effects is remarkably small. In most cases recovery is complete.

At times, symptoms such as headache, dizziness, irritability, etc., persist following an injury (post-traumatic or post-concussion syndrome). These do not, as a rule, indicate any serious underlying disorder or complication. It must be realized that there is a strong emotional component to every physical injury, and this is particularly true when the accident has involved the head. Psychological disturbances and emotional instability after skull and brain injuries can often be minimized by careful explanation of the exact nature of the injury. Above all, it is important to assure such patients that their ability to return to a completely normal life need not be impaired when they have recovered fully from the physical effects of the accident.

SURGICAL INFECTIONS OF
THE SKULL AND BRAIN

Do all types of infection of the skull or brain require surgical treatment?

No. Surgery is not indicated in cases in which the infection is widespread (encephalitis, meningitis) and in which there is no localized collection of pus to drain.

How does the brain or its coverings become infected?

Sinusitis and, less often, injury are the most common causes of infection of the bones of the skull (osteomyelitis). An abscess within the brain occurs as a result of the spread of an infection from an adjacent structure such as the sinuses or ears, or from a distant part of the body, usually the lung. It may also be caused by a penetrating wound of the skull or by a compound skull fracture.

Is osteomyelitis of the skull serious?

Yes. Unless it is adequately treated, there is danger of the spread of infection to the brain. This type of infection is encountered less often than in the days before the advent of chemotherapy and antibiotics.

What does the surgical treatment of osteomyelitis entail?

Removal of the diseased bone and provision for drainage of pus. Antibiotics are administered concurrently.

How serious is a brain abscess?

Brain abscess is a very serious condition, despite the fact that its incidence has diminished markedly and the outlook for successful treatment has improved considerably as a result of the introduction of chemotherapy and antibiotics. It is treated by surgical excision or drainage.

TUMORS OF THE BRAIN

How common are tumors of the brain?

The brain is one of the most frequent sites of tumor formation in the entire body.

Are there different kinds of brain tumors?

Yes. The term intracranial tumor is used to denote any one of several types of growths which may be present within the skull. A tumor may originate from the skull, from the membranes or nerves external to the brain, or from the brain itself. Still another source of origin is the pituitary gland at the base of the skull. Finally, cancerous growths arising elsewhere in the body may spread by means of the bloodstream to involve the brain secondarily.

What determines the outlook in a particular case of brain tumor?

The nature of the growth and its location. Tumors arising from the coverings of the brain (meningiomas) and the nerves of the brain (neurofibromas), when surgically accessible, may be completely removed and the patient cured. As these tumors represent 20 per cent of all growths within the skull, it is obvious that many patients can look forward to complete recovery.

Pituitary gland tumors, in a high proportion of cases, may be successfully treated by means of x-ray alone, without resorting to surgery. Those patients not helped by x-ray treatment can subsequently be benefited by surgery. Pituitary tumors constitute about 10 per cent of all brain tumors.

Approximately 50 per cent of brain tumors develop within the brain substance itself (gliomas). With few exceptions, these tumors are not sufficiently well localized to be removed completely. Their rate of growth varies, being exceedingly rapid in the more malignant varieties. Some may grow slowly over a period of years, while others may go on to a rapid termination within a much shorter time. Even when complete cure cannot be accomplished, many people with this type of brain tumor can be helped by surgery. However, a brain tumor incompletely removed eventually recurs, and the ultimate outlook depends upon its rate of growth. The growth of some of these tumors is retarded by x-ray treatment, which is therefore often carried out after surgery.

Occasionally, the position of a tumor is such that the surgeon is unable to approach it directly without risking serious consequences or even the life of the patient. In such cases, an operation for the reduction of intracranial pressure may be accomplished with relative safety and may bring relief of symptoms for a variable period of time.

What are the chances of surviving an operation for brain tumor?

Eighty-five to 90 per cent.

What are the most common symptoms of brain tumor?

Headache, vomiting, disturbances of vision, and various specific symptoms, depending on the location of the tumor, such as paralysis or convulsions.

What causes brain tumors?

As in the case of tumors elsewhere in the body, the cause is unknown.

Are brain tumors hereditary?

No.

Can the exact location of a brain tumor be determined before operation?

In most instances, yes.

How is the location of a brain tumor determined?

A detailed history and a careful examination of the patient may yield important clues. As a rule, however, it is desirable, and at times necessary, to perform some of the following diagnostic procedures in order to establish the location of a tumor:

a. Plain x-rays of the skull. These may yield sufficient information.

b. Examination of the spinal fluid.

c. Examination of the eyes (visual fields).

d. Encephalograms or ventriculograms are often necessary. In performing these tests, some of the fluid surrounding the brain and contained within its cavities is removed through a needle and is replaced with a gas (helium or oxygen). The gas, acting as a contrast medium, outlines the chambers of the brain on an x-ray film. Familiarity with the normal appearance of these cavities permits one to recognize the distortion produced by a tumor and to identify its location.

e. Arteriograms, by outlining the blood vessels of the brain, may provide valuable information. By injecting a radio-opaque substance into the arteries of the neck, the blood vessels of the brain can be visualized on an x-ray film. A brain tumor, by concentrating the radio-opaque substance within its own blood vessels, may actually be outlined. In other instances, its location may be revealed by noting the displacement of the blood vessels of the brain from their normal position.

f. Electroencephalography, the study of the electrical brain waves, is another valuable diagnostic test. It is often possible to record abnormal brain waves from the scalp over an area corresponding to the site of a brain tumor.

Is it possible to determine before operation whether a brain tumor is benign or malignant?

Not in all cases, though at times one can be reasonably certain.

What kind of anesthesia is used for brain surgery?

Either local or general anesthesia, preferably the latter, through a tube placed into the trachea (windpipe).

Where are the incisions made in cases of brain surgery?

Over any part of the scalp, depending on the location of the underlying condition.

Is the scar resulting from brain surgery disfiguring?

No. Insofar as possible, the incisions are made within the hairline, and the eventual scar is inconspicuous.

Are blood transfusions administered during the course of brain operations?

Yes, very often.

How long do brain operations take to perform?

The time element varies, depending on the nature of the condition requiring surgery, and the procedure to be performed. Some operations can be completed within an hour or two; others may require four to five hours.

Can patients safely withstand this type of surgery for several hours?

Yes. Improved anesthetic techniques and supportive measures make it possible for lengthy operations to be performed safely.

How soon after a major brain operation can the surgeon tell if the patient will survive?

Usually, within a few days.

Are special nurses necessary after brain operations?

Yes, for several days.

How long a hospital stay is necessary after a major brain operation?

About two weeks.

Must one take special care of the wound area after a brain operation has been performed?

Not usually. The only cases which require special attention are those in which the piece of bone removed at operation has not been replaced.

Do brain tumors, once removed, tend to recur?

Only if incompletely removed.

Can a patient who has had a brain tumor successfully removed live a normal life?

Yes.

Do brain tumors occur in children?

Yes. Brain tumors during childhood are not at all uncommon. Certain types of tumors are especially prevalent in children and they tend to occur predominantly in certain locations within the brain. Both benign and malignant varieties are encountered. Their treatment is similar to that of tumors in adults and the results obtained are comparable. Children withstand brain surgery as well as adults.

Is x-ray treatment rather than surgery ever recommended for brain tumors?

Yes. X-ray treatment is effective in a high proportion of tumors of the pituitary gland.

If vision is lost because of a brain condition, does it ever return?

If vision is lost as a result of increased pressure within the skull, the outlook for recovery is not good. In cases in which vision is damaged, surgery may prevent further impairment or result in improvement. Loss of vision due to direct pressure of the tumor on the optic nerves may be helped considerably through surgery.

If hearing is lost because of a brain tumor, is it ever regained after surgical removal?

A brain tumor causing loss of hearing usually arises from the auditory nerve and hearing will not return despite the removal of the tumor.

Can a patient who has lost the power to speak be taught to speak again after removal of a brain tumor?

Yes. Very often this is possible with intensive effort and training.

Can patients regain the use of their limbs following removal of a brain tumor?

Yes, in many cases. Complete recovery, however, does not always take place.

Is a patient's mentality usually affected by a brain operation?

As a rule, no. The patient's mental reaction is primarily determined by the nature and location of the disease from which he is suffering.

Will the removal of a brain tumor result in a cessation of convulsions?

The frequency of the convulsions may be diminished, but they are not always eliminated completely. Hence, the administration of anticonvulsant medication should be continued following operation. Even in cases in which convulsions did not occur preoperatively, the use of anticonvulsant medication postoperatively is advisable as a precautionary measure.

INTRACRANIAL HEMORRHAGE

What is meant by cerebral hemorrhage?

Bleeding occurring within the substance of the brain or on its surface.

What are the common causes of cerebral hemorrhage?

a. Hardening of the arteries (arteriosclerosis) and high blood pressure are the most common causes of hemorrhage within the brain. This type of hemorrhage usually occurs after the age of forty.

919

b. Bleeding may also take place in younger individuals as a result of rupture of a malformed blood vessel. Most often, the malformation is a sac-like dilatation of a blood vessel (aneurysm). Occasionally, it consists of a cluster of abnormally large blood vessels (angioma).

c. Injury to the brain may also cause intracranial hemorrhage.

Is a cerebral hemorrhage synonymous with a stroke?

Not entirely. The term "stroke" includes several conditions, one of which is cerebral hemorrhage.

Is cerebral hemorrhage serious?

Yes, regardless of cause.

What is the role of surgery in the treatment of cerebral hemorrhage?

Hemorrhage within the brain, when it is caused by rupture of a diseased or abnormal blood vessel, sometimes lends itself to surgical treatment. Operation may, in certain cases, be a lifesaving measure and may lessen the likelihood of permanent brain damage.

What is the role of surgery in the treatment of malformation of the intracranial blood vessels?

Because these deformed vessels often rupture and cause intracranial bleeding, they constitute a threat to life. Obviously, it would be desirable to discover them and, wherever possible, to institute treatment *before* they cause hemorrhage. Unfortunately, evidence of hemorrhage is often the first indication of their presence. The use of radio-opaque substances in order to outline the blood vessels of the brain (arteriography) is especially useful in cases in which an abnormality of the blood vessels is suspected.

Various methods of surgical treatment have been devised to deal with abnormalities of the intracranial blood vessels, but, unfortunately, such operations are not always feasible.

❊   ❊   ❊   ❊

What is meant by trigeminal neuralgia (tic douloureux, trifacial neuralgia)?

Trigeminal neuralgia is a disease occurring mostly in middle-aged and elderly people, characterized by severe, recurrent paroxysmal pain in the face. Its cause is unknown.

What is the treatment of trigeminal neuralgia?

There is no medication which is dependable in affording relief. Injection of alcohol into the nerves in the face may eliminate the pain for periods of varying duration. Cutting the main nerve within the skull responsible for the pain, provides permanent relief. This operation is successful in the great majority of cases.

Is surgery ever indicated in the treatment of epilepsy?

Yes, though relatively infrequently. Epilepsy may occur in the absence of any demonstrable cause (idiopathic), or may result from the presence of some structural abnormality in the brain, such as a tumor, abscess, blood vessel malformation, or scar. It is essential to differentiate the idiopathic cases from those due to a known organic disease. The cause of idiopathic epilepsy is unknown and treatment is designed exclusively for the purpose of controlling the seizures. Medication is employed in the management of this type of case.

An entirely different problem is presented by the patient whose seizures are not idiopathic in nature. Control of the seizures must still be achieved, but, in addition, the underlying condition must also be treated. It is this type of case that may require surgical treatment. Thus, an operation is indicated if the basic condition is a tumor, abscess, or depressed fracture. Surgery may be advisable in cases of epilepsy due to scar formation, if the seizures cannot be effectively controlled by medication. Certain patients with uncontrollable psychomotor epilepsy, characterized by the performance of some sort of automatic activity during a period of amnesia, may also be benefited by surgery.

What is the role of surgery in the treatment of mental disease?

Brain surgery for the treatment of chronic mental illness consists of an operation performed in the frontal region of the brain. This procedure is known as a lobotomy. Its purpose is to cut the connecting nerve fibers between certain areas of the brain. The selection of patients with mental disorders for operation is primarily a function of the psychiatrist. In general, surgery is recommended for patients

921

whose outlook is otherwise very poor. The results are most favorable in the psychoneurotic disorders (obsessive compulsive neurosis, hypochondriasis) and in the affective psychoses characterized by disturbance of mood (involutional and manic depressive psychosis). Improvement may also occur in paranoid psychoses and certain types of dementia praecox. The favorable effects of lobotomy include a reduction of anxiety, fear, assaultiveness, agitation, and self-concern. Less desirable personality changes, such as apathy, impaired judgment, loss of initiative, and lack of inhibition, must also be anticipated.

Generally speaking, the enthusiasm for lobotomy has dwindled considerably in recent years, and, since the introduction of the so-called tranquilizing drugs into the field of psychiatry, the operation is performed relatively infrequently today.

Is surgery of value in the treatment of Parkinsonism(shaking palsy)?

Yes. Recently, the region of the brain that must be cut to relieve the palsy without causing paralysis, has been quite clearly defined. As a result, many patients who formerly had to be treated solely by medication, can now be helped greatly by surgery. The tremor and rigidity characteristic of this disease can be relieved in a great many instances.

What is meant by hydrocephalus?

Hydrocephalus is a relatively common disorder of infants in which the head enlarges abnormally because of an excessive amount of cerebrospinal fluid within the brain. Interference with the circulation or absorption of cerebrospinal fluid is responsible for an excessive accumulation. The size of the head may reach enormous proportions.

What is the treatment of hydrocephalus?

Spontaneous arrest occurs infrequently, so that various surgical procedures have been devised in an attempt to deal with this condition. Unfortunately, the results are not invariably satisfactory. An operation may be performed, either for the purpose of reducing the formation of fluid or in order to lead the fluid outside its normal channels in the nervous system; the effect in either case being to lower the intracranial pressure. Insufficient time has elapsed to evaluate the effectiveness of the more recent types of operation.

SPINAL CORD

BIRTH DEFORMITIES

(Congenital Malformations, Developmental Anomalies)

What are the common malformations involving the spinal cord?

Incomplete closure of some part of the vertebral canal is a fairly common developmental deformity and usually causes no symptoms (spina bifida occulta). It may, however, be associated with a protrusion or herniation of the membranes covering the spinal cord. Such a protrusion may contain cerebrospinal fluid only (meningocele), or it may contain nerve elements and even part of the spinal cord itself (meningomyelocele).

How does a meningocele or meningomyelocele manifest itself?

Infants with these conditions are born with a noticeable lump on the back. Inclusion of nerve structures in the malformation usually is accompanied by varying degrees of paralysis of the lower limbs.

Can a child be born with more than one malformation?

Yes. Hydrocephalus often occurs or develops in association with a meningocele.

Can anything be done to remedy a developmental defect (meningocele, meningomyelocele)?

Nothing can be done to correct an existing paralysis. Operation is performed solely for the purpose of repairing the deformity. Occasionally, in cases in which the sac is very thin and threatens to rupture, surgery may be required soon after birth.

923

TUMORS OF THE SPINAL CORD

What are the usual symptoms resulting from a tumor of the spinal cord?

Backache, together with weakness and numbness of the limbs, and disturbances referable to the bladder and bowels.

Are there different kinds of tumors of the spinal cord?

Yes. The spinal cord may be affected by tumors compressing it from without or growing within its substance. About 50 per cent of these tumors originate from the membranes overlying the cord or from a spinal nerve.

How is the diagnosis of a spinal cord tumor established?

The presence of a spinal cord tumor may be suspected on the basis of the history and examination of the patient. Spinal puncture usually reveals an obstruction to the free flow of cerebrospinal fluid. Examination of the spinal fluid often provides useful information. The diagnosis may be further confirmed by introducing a radio-opaque substance into the cerebrospinal fluid and subjecting the patient to fluoroscopy. This procedure is called myelography. Normally, the radio-opaque substance flows freely when the patient is tilted in either direction. A tumor will act as an obstruction to the flow of the radio-opaque substance, thus verifying the diagnosis and providing evidence of its exact location.

What are the results of surgery in the treatment of spinal cord tumors?

Tumors originating from the membranes overlying the spinal cord or from a spinal nerve can usually be totally removed and the patient cured or greatly improved. If the spinal cord damage has been unduly prolonged, it may be irreversible. Tumors growing within the substance of the spinal cord usually cannot be removed, but their growth can often be halted by x-ray treatment. Not infrequently, a cancer which has originated in some other part of the body spreads to involve the spinal cord. The outlook in such cases is especially poor, though x-ray treatment, and occasionally surgery, may prove temporarily beneficial.

Can paralysis caused by a spinal cord tumor be relieved by surgery?

Yes. In about 50 per cent of all cases, the tumor can be removed completely and the patient cured or improved without fear of recurrence of the tumor.

Are operations upon the spinal cord dangerous?

No more so than a major operation elsewhere in the body.

What kind of anesthesia is used when operating upon the spinal cord?

General anesthesia, as a rule, administered through a tube in the trachea (windpipe).

RUPTURED INTERVERTEBRAL DISCS
(Herniated, Slipped Discs)

What is a ruptured disc?

Intervertebral discs are elastic structures interposed between adjacent vertebrae. As a result of degeneration and injury, a disc may protrude into the spinal canal and give rise to pain. Ruptured discs occur most frequently in the lower back and give rise to backache and pain radiating down the leg. Less frequently the protrusion occurs in the neck, in which case the pain is located in the neck and upper limb.

How is the diagnosis of a ruptured disc established?

The diagnosis may be strongly suspected on the basis of the history of the patient and physical examination. Plain x-rays of the spine may or may not provide additional useful information. Myelography (x-rays outlining the spinal canal) usually resolves all doubt as to diagnosis.

What is the treatment of a ruptured disc?

Conservative measures, such as bed rest, traction, and physiotherapy, are worth a trial in the treatment of this condition. Should pain and disability persist after a reasonable period of conservative treatment or should there be recurrent attacks, operation is indicated.

925

Are disc operations dangerous?

No.

Is it necessary to fuse the spine after a disc operation?

Only in a very small proportion of cases.

How long a hospital stay is required for a disc operation?

About seven to ten days.

How successful are operations for ruptured disc?

About 85 per cent of patients are completely or considerably relieved of pain.

Do ruptured discs ever recur?

They may, though infrequently.

Does the removal of a ruptured disc ever result in paralysis?

No.

Does removal of a ruptured disc affect one's sex life?

No.

SPINAL CORD INJURIES

What are the common causes of spinal cord injury?

Injuries of the spinal cord usually occur in association with fractures or dislocations of the spinal column. Falls, automobile and driving accidents, and gunshot wounds are the most frequent causes. The spinal cord may escape injury at the time a spinal fracture is incurred, but careless transportation of the patient from the scene of the accident may result in damage to the spinal cord.

How does a spinal cord injury manifest itself?

The manifestations of spinal cord injury include varying degrees of paralysis, loss of sensation, and inability to control the bladder and bowels.

What is the outlook for recovery following spinal cord injury?

In cases in which there is a complete paralysis and loss of all forms of sensation, the outlook for recovery is very poor. The retention of some degree of spinal cord function, no matter how slight, renders the outlook infinitely better than when all function is lost. If evidence of complete interruption of the spinal cord persists for more than one week, it is unlikely that any improvement will occur. Regeneration of divided fibers does not occur in the spinal cord.

Is surgery of value in the treatment of spinal cord injury?

In most cases of spinal cord injury, operation is useless. There are occasional exceptions, but, as a rule, all that can be accomplished is to institute orthopedic measures to treat the spinal fracture or dislocation.

Is there any hope for the patient who remains paralyzed?

The management of the patient who remains paralyzed is a complex problem beyond the scope of this discussion. Suffice it to say, after prolonged training it is possible to rehabilitate many of these unfortunate paraplegics so that they can be made ambulatory and lead a reasonably normal and useful life again.

SURGERY FOR INTRACTABLE PAIN

Are operations on the spinal cord performed for the relief of pain?

Yes. The neurosurgeon is often called upon to relieve pain which fails to respond to medication. Such pain is usually caused by advanced cancer. The location of the pathways within the spinal cord conducting pain being known, it is possible to cut them and afford the patient relief. This type of operation is known as a cordotomy.

It is also possible to cut the nerves (as they enter the spinal cord) which supply a particular region of the body. By depriving that area of all sensation, pain is eliminated. This procedure is called a rhizotomy.

Both of these operations upon the spinal cord are safe procedures, and although they do not cure the underlying condition, in suitable cases they are extremely valuable for the relief of intractable pain.

927

Does an operation upon the spinal cord for the relief of pain (cordotomy) result in paralysis?

No.

PERIPHERAL NERVES

What is a peripheral nerve?

One which conveys impulses between the spinal cord and some other part of the body. It may transmit impulses concerned with muscular contraction as well as stimuli conveying sensory impressions.

How do nerve injuries occur?

They may occur as a result of blunt trauma, punctures, lacerations, incisions, or penetrating (gunshot or stab) wounds.

Where do peripheral nerve injuries occur most commonly?

In the limbs.

What are the symptoms of peripheral nerve injury?

Paralysis of the muscles and loss of sensation over a specific area supplied by that particular nerve.

What is the role of surgery in the treatment of peripheral nerve injuries?

Nerves are capable of regrowth and resumption of function provided the cut ends are accurately united. This is precisely what the surgeon seeks to accomplish at operation. A good result is not always achieved following surgery, however, even under optimum conditions, and at times additional corrective orthopedic measures are necessary. Physiotherapy is an important adjunct in the treatment of this type of case.

Is surgery necessary in all types of nerve injury?

No; only in cases in which a nerve has been severed.

Can tumors arise from peripheral nerves?

Yes. Fortunately, such tumors are usually benign and can be removed completely.

43 *The Newborn Child*

How can it be determined that a newborn child is normal?

This is usually the first question asked of a pediatrician. It can be answered only after a thorough examination of the newborn baby. This should always be done within the first few days of life. Many of the little abnormalities found within the first few days will disappear spontaneously and should cause no concern.

Do newborn babies ever display slight difficulty in breathing?

Yes. At birth, there may be an excessive collection of mucus in the baby's throat. The nursery nurse will suction this out and thus improve the baby's breathing.

Why does a newborn baby's head sometimes have a peculiar shape?

The elongated or irregular shape of the baby's head is caused by "molding" which takes place during the birth of the baby. The head will usually return to its normal shape in one to three weeks, although it may take longer in some instances.

Is there a chance of injuring the "soft spot" (fontanelle) on the baby's head?

No. This area is rarely injured, and ordinary washing and touching will not hurt it.

May a newborn child's head be washed?

Yes.

Why do some newborns have an egg-shaped swelling on the head?

This may occur because of bleeding beneath the skin of the scalp as a result of pressure during passage down the birth canal. It does not extend into the skull, does not involve the brain, and will be slowly absorbed, leaving no after-effects.

Is it significant if a baby is born with very little hair?

No. Many babies are born with very little hair; others will lose some of the hair they do have. Baby hair may fall out, but new hair will grow in later. There may even be some fine, downy hair on the body or forehead. This, too, will disappear in a short time.

What special care is needed for the baby's scalp?

Wash the scalp with soap and water two or three times a week. Use baby oil at other times. This prevents the formation of scalp crusts or "cradle cap." If cradle cap forms, it can be washed thoroughly and combed out with a fine comb. In some instances your doctor will give you a salve to be applied to the scalp to prevent the re-formation of this crust.

What care should be given to the baby's eyes, ears, and mouth?

It is not necessary to wash the baby's eyes and ears, or to cleanse the nose or mouth. Nature has provided fluids and secretions for cleansing them without any outside assistance. If any wax accumulates on the outside of the ears, it may be washed away gently, but do not poke into the ear canals.

Does anything need to be done about a short membrane (frenum) under the baby's tongue?

In most instances nothing needs to be done, particularly if the baby can protrude the tongue adequately. This so-called "tongue-tie" does not affect speech or produce any lisp. The old practice of clipping this membrane is no longer followed, except when it is

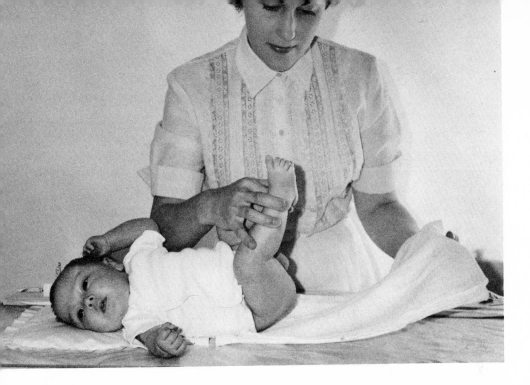

Diapering the Baby.   Infants differ considerably in the number of diapers they require during the course of a day. It is important for mothers to determine that the soaps or detergents used in washing diapers are not irritating to the delicate skin of the infant.

An infant will usually let it be known when the diaper is soiled. When putting on a diaper, care should be taken not to prick the fingers with the safety pin, as a severe infection can result therefrom.

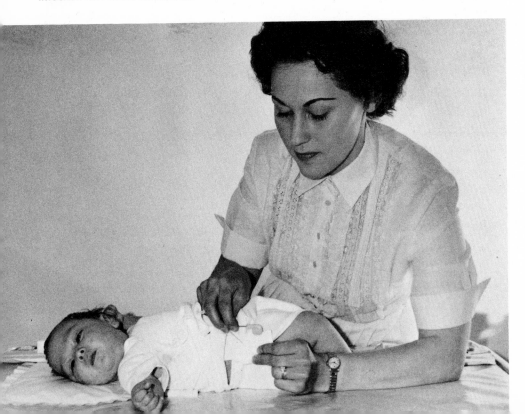

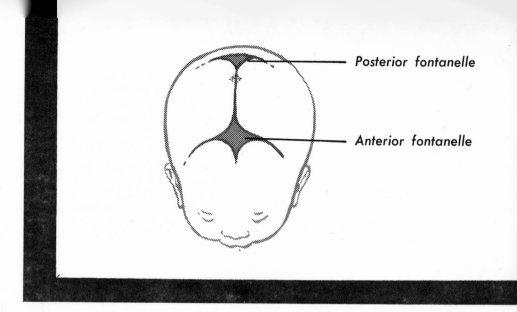

Open Fontanelles of the Skull of the Newborn Child. These apertures between the bones of the skull usually take a year or longer to fill in. Contrary to common belief, injuries to these areas are very rare.

very thick, very short, or actually affects the ability of the baby to protrude the tongue beyond the lip margins.

Why do some babies have a slightly yellow color (jaundice)?

Many babies will develop this light yellow skin color about the third to fifth day of life. This is normal and nothing needs to be done about it. It will disappear spontaneously in about seven to ten days. This is called physiologic jaundice. If jaundice appears earlier, or is more intense, or increases instead of disappearing, it will require the attention of your doctor for diagnosis and treatment.

What are the many small red spots on the baby's skin, seen during the first few days of life?

These are a reaction to the amniotic fluid which surrounded the baby in the womb. They will disappear in a few days.

Why does the newborn infant's skin peel?

After having been in a fluid environment for nine months, some infants' skin will peel. The skin is very sensitive at this stage and may react to rubbing, washing, warmth, or irritation of clothing. The reaction may cause some redness or peeling of the skin.

What is the meaning of small pus pimples on the abdomen or in the groin?

This is the result of a skin infection called impetigo of the newborn. It will clear readily with antibiotic ointments or washing with an antiseptic soap. In some cases antibiotics may also be used internally.

What is the meaning of a bluish spot at the base of the spine?

This spot has no significance and will disappear in time, perhaps within a year. Similar spots may be present over the buttocks. No treatment is necessary.

Why do babies lose weight during the first few days of life?

All mothers seem to be concerned about this early loss of weight, yet it occurs with every newborn baby. In breast-fed infants it occurs because the milk does not appear in the mother's breast until the third or fourth day after delivery. In bottle-fed babies, it occurs because of the very small amounts of formula fed to the baby.

What is the reason for the eye drops given to newborn babies?

Practically all communities require that some antiseptic be instilled into a baby's eyes as soon as it is born, to prevent the possible spread of any infection from the mother's vagina. In some states, silver nitrate is used. In other places, it is permissible to use a few drops of penicillin solution or some other antibiotic. Such drops will prevent a gonorrheal eye infection if the mother is affected with this disease.

What is the meaning of the marks over the baby's eyes?

Some babies are born with small pressure marks on the eyelids, on the forehead, and over the back of the neck. These have no significance and will usually disappear in a few weeks, though occasionally they may last several months.

Will the color of the baby's eyes change?

The color of the eyes at birth will not be the final color. It usually takes up to six months for the final color to be established.

933

When does a newborn learn to focus his eyes?

At about two to three months of age.

Is it natural for a newborn's eyes to appear crossed?

Yes. Not all newborns can make their eyes synchronize perfectly during the first year of life. Do not conclude that the baby's eyes are crossed until such a condition persists beyond the age of one to one and a half years.

Why do some babies have small blood spots in their eyes?

These spots are caused by tiny hemorrhages in the conjunctiva or covering of the eyeball and will disappear without leaving any after-effects.

Does the puffiness of the baby's eyes have any significance?

No. This, too, is temporary.

Why does the baby have some discharge from the eyes on the second or third day?

The discharge is usually caused by the drops that were instilled at birth. It will disappear within a few days.

Why are the baby's breasts swollen?

Most babies, boys and girls alike, have some swelling of the breasts at birth or soon thereafter. This is caused by a hormone which was circulating through both the mother's and baby's bloodstreams. It is the hormone which induces the production of milk in the mother's breasts.

What treatment is necessary for swollen breasts?

None, unless the breasts become red, inflamed, and tender. The swelling and any milk secretion will subside without treatment.

Why do some babies have small white spots on their noses?

These are due to collections of skin oil which have not been able to escape from the oil glands. Usually the surface film will come off in the washing and the white oil collections will disappear.

Is it necessary to circumcise a male infant?

Circumcision is practiced by some people as a religious ritual. Nowadays, it is advised by most physicians for all babies in order to safeguard cleanliness in the area of the penis. Also, the incidence of cancer of the penis is practically nil if circumcision has been carried out in infancy. However, circumcision is not medically essential if the foreskin can be pulled back easily over the head of the penis.

When can a circumcision be done?

In cases where it is done as a ritual procedure, the circumcision is usually done on the eighth day of life. It may, however, be done safely on the third or fourth day of life. In some hospitals, the obstetrician will perform circumcision as soon as the baby is born. It is essential that the baby's bleeding time be determined prior to circumcision in order to uncover any abnormal bleeding tendency and to avoid possible postoperative hemorrhage.

What care should be given after circumcision?

The bandages may be removed in two to three days. Apply warm, sterile, water dressings around the penis several times daily after painting the affected area with 2 per cent mercurochrome solution. Later, apply sterile vaseline to prevent sticking of the gauze.

Does the rectal area need any special handling?

No. Just wash gently with soap and water, as any other part of the body.

Does the vaginal area need any special handling?

No. Just the ordinary cleansing, preferably with a motion going from the vaginal area backward toward the rectal area.

Will a hernia result if the umbilical cord was tied off long?

The umbilical cord is usually tied off about one to two inches from the baby's body. This entire area will dry up and fall off in about a week, leaving a moist area of healing. This, in turn, will dry and heal a few days later. The length of the tied cord will not influence development of a hernia.

935

What care should be given after the cord has fallen off?

The area should be cleansed with a little alcohol, applied on a cotton applicator, twice a day, until it is completely healed. This will take about a week or ten days. If there is a little bleeding, don't be disturbed by it. Occasionally, a small area of "proudflesh" may be found remaining at the navel. This can be cauterized by the baby's physician and will then heal promptly.

Is an abdominal binder or bellyband necessary?

No. These do not help in the healing of the cord, nor do they prevent a rupture or hernia from forming. Only a dry, clean gauze dressing needs to be applied to the area while it is healing.

What is the significance of swelling of the scrotum?

In most cases it is caused by an accumulation of fluid. This condition is called a hydrocele. The majority of hydroceles in newborns disappear by themselves within a year after birth.

It is, however, important for your physician to examine all swellings in the scrotum to make sure that a hernia (rupture) is not present.

Can crying cause a hernia in a boy baby?

No. Hernia is a developmental defect present at birth.

Why do some newborn baby's legs appear bowed?

This is due to the position in which the legs were crossed in the uterus. This bowing will disappear in time without treatment.

How soon may the baby have a sponge bath?

As soon as the baby is taken home from the hospital.

How soon may the baby have a tub bath?

As soon as the umbilical area has healed completely. In the case of a male baby who has been circumcised, it is wise to wait until the circumcision area is healed too. This will usually take about seven to ten days.

At what temperature should the baby's room be kept?

Seventy to 72°F., during the day; 65° to 68°F., at night. A room that is too warm is just as harmful as one that is too cold. Always be sure there is some air entering the room, and avoid the use of kerosene or gas stoves in the room for heating purposes.

When may the baby be taken out of doors?

About seven to ten days after the mother leaves the hospital, providing that the weather is good. Start with a quarter-hour the first day, a half-hour the second day, and so on. Don't take the baby out if the weather is very cold (below 40°F.), windy, or damp. Be sure the baby is adequately protected from the direct glare of the sun.

Does a baby have to be taken out of doors every day?

No. Fresh air from an open window is just as healthful. Avoid going out in bad weather.

When should visitors be permitted to see the new baby?

It is best to keep all visitors away from the newborn for the first week or two of life. Certainly, anyone (including the mother) with a cold or sore throat should be kept away. After this period, healthy people may be allowed to see and hold the baby, preferably just before bath time.

Can a newborn baby be given a pacifier if he cries excessively?

Yes. If it is found to satisfy him, it does no harm.

Why must newborn babies be viewed through a glass window?

To prevent germs or infection from reaching the babies.

May pictures of the newborn baby be taken with a flash bulb?

Yes. The flash bulb will not in any way affect the baby's eyes.

PREMATURE BABIES

What is meant by a premature baby?

Ordinarily, any baby born before term (nine months) is considered premature. Because we are not sure of the exact length of pregnancy in all cases, all babies who weigh less than five and one-half pounds are considered premature and are treated accordingly.

Do premature babies tend to have more defects than other newborns?

Yes. However, the great majority are structurally normal.

What special care is required for premature babies?

Most premature babies are best cared for in a hospital where special facilities are available. They may require an incubator or a heated crib. Special formulas must be made, and feedings are often given by tube or dropper.

When can a premature baby leave the hospital?

If the baby is thriving, he may be taken home when he weighs about five and one-half pounds.

What are the chances for survival of a premature baby?

The smaller and less mature the baby, the less are his chances of survival. However, many more babies are being saved today than ever before. A baby over four or four and one-half pounds has an excellent chance, if there are no defects in his heart, brain, or lungs. Babies between four and five and one-half pounds have a 75 per cent or better chance of survival. Those between three and four pounds have better than a 50 per cent chance, but those below three pounds have a considerably poorer chance.

What chance does a two- to three-pound baby have?

Very little chance. The mortality rate in this weight group is about 60 to 70 per cent.

Does a baby under two pounds have any chance?

Occasionally, such a baby may survive, but it has only a 5 per cent chance.

Does the length of the pregnancy have anything to do with survival rate?

Yes. The longer the pregnancy, the better the chances of the baby's survival.

If a baby is carried to full term but weighs very little, will he have a better chance than a premature baby of equal weight?

Yes.

Is it true that seven-month babies have a better chance than eight-month babies?

No. This is a common misconception.

Is oxygen supplied to every premature baby?

No. It is supplied only when necessary for the respiration of the premature baby and then only in a special concentration and only for a few days. It has been found that excessive use of oxygen may be harmful to the baby's eyes.

How long does the baby stay in an incubator?

As long as it needs the added oxygen or warmth.

Are the cribs heated for premature babies?

Some of the open-air cribs are heated and used when the baby is removed from the incubator.

Can a premature baby be transported from home to hospital, or from hospital to hospital?

Yes. There are special ambulances that have portable incubators. These supply heat and oxygen to the baby while he is being transported.

Can any hospital care for a premature infant?

The larger prematures can be treated in any hospital, but the smaller ones require the special facilities that are present in what are called "Premature Centers."

Is the premature baby fed right after birth?

No. Usually a wait of a day or longer is advised.

Can a premature baby suck from a nipple?

The larger prematures can, but not the smaller ones.

How are the smaller premature infants fed?

A polyethylene tube is inserted through the nose into the baby's gullet and then down into the stomach. Small amounts of formula are then "fed" into the stomach by way of this tube.

Can the feeding tube stay in the stomach for several days?

Yes.

How long is the tube kept in place?

Until the baby can suck from a nipple. This may take several days or weeks.

Is this tube harmful or painful if kept in for prolonged periods?

No.

What amounts are fed the baby?

At the start, as little as a half teaspoon (2cc.) at a time. Such feedings may be given every hour or two. The amounts are increased very slowly, depending upon the baby's tolerance and weight gain.

Does the premature baby require any special dietary supplements?

Yes. Vitamins may be given earlier and iron drops may be added to the milk because the premature baby has not been able to store a supply of vitamins and iron which he would have normally received from his mother during the last month or two of uterine development. Also, small amounts of calcium are sometimes added to the baby's diet.

Is there a tendency for a premature baby to be anemic?

Yes, and he may remain so for several weeks or months.

What other treatments are given to premature babies?

Some babies require additional fluid by vein or under the skin if they cannot absorb sufficient quantities through the stomach tube.

Are transfusions ever required by premature babies?

Rarely. However, if the hemoglobin is very low, it may be necessary to give a blood transfusion. Most prematures will respond satisfactorily to iron supplements in the diet.

Are premature babies ever given antibiotics?

Yes. In some hospitals, antibiotics are given routinely to prevent secondary infections, to which such babies may be prone.

Are prematures given routine baths and similar care?

It is usually advisable not to handle them too much, although the skin must be watched very carefully.

Is any special care given to the eyes or ears of the premature baby?

Usually not. Their eyes should be examined about once a week to determine any evidence of disturbance.

Does prematurity affect the baby's heart or lungs?

Not ordinarily, although premature babies are more susceptible to a rare lung condition known as hyaline membrane disease.

Will prematurity affect the baby's later mental development?

If there are no organic brain defects at birth, the premature baby, with good care, should develop normally after he has been discharged from the hospital. In some cases he may be a little slower in his early development, but he will catch up by completion of the first year of life.

The Nose

44

and Sinuses

What is the structure and function of the nose?

The nose is made up of bone and cartilage and contains two cavities which are separated by a septum. The nose acts as a natural airway for respiration; it acts as an air conditioner, by filtering, moistening, and warming the air which is breathed in; and it functions as the organ of smell. Also, the hairs within the nose prevent dust from gaining access to the throat, and a mucus which lines the membrane of the nose further settles out dust and bacteria, thus protecting against infection.

FRACTURED NOSE

Is fracture of the nose a frequent occurrence?

Yes. It is one of the most common injuries, because of the exposed position of the structure and because the nasal bones are thin and delicate.

Does bleeding from the nose always take place with a fracture?

Yes.

Should x-rays be taken to determine nasal fracture?

If there is no doubt about the diagnosis, it may not be necessary to take x-rays. However, x-rays must be taken after a fracture has

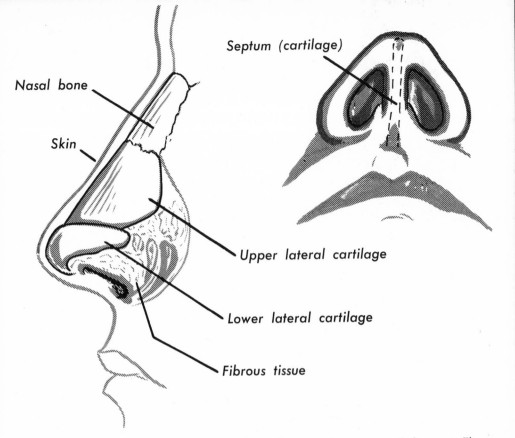

Nasal bone

Skin

Septum (cartilage)

Upper lateral cartilage

Lower lateral cartilage

Fibrous tissue

Anatomy of the Nose. This diagram shows the normal anatomy of the nose. The bones in the nose are quite fragile and fracture occurs frequently. Fortunately, the nose can be restored to its normal shape without too much difficulty.

been set, in order to make sure that the fragments are in proper alignment.

How soon after a nasal fracture occurs should it be treated?

As soon as possible, preferably within a few hours, for at this time manipulation of the fragments and setting of the fracture can be accomplished easily. After the passage of several days, it is much more difficult to bring a nose back into proper alignment.

What methods are used to set a fractured nose?

a. Manipulation by the hand of the surgeon, externally.
b. Insertion of special instruments into the nasal cavity to push out depressed bony fragments.

Is it necessary to use anesthesia to set a nasal fracture?

Most cases can be set under local anesthesia, but when the pain is too great a general anesthetic agent should be used.

Is hospitalization necessary for a fracture of the nose?

Only if there is an extensive or compound fracture, or if general anesthesia is necessary, or if there are accompanying injuries which require hospitalization.

How long does it take a fracture of the nose to heal?

These are very rapidly healing fractures, because of the rich blood supply in the nasal area. Healing usually takes place within two to three weeks.

How long does the swelling of the nose persist after a fracture?

Slight swelling may continue for several months, but the greatest part will subside in two to three weeks.

Are antibiotics used following the setting of a nasal fracture?

Yes, to minimize the danger of infection.

Is a fracture of the nose usually followed by a permanent deformity?

No. However, there may be some thickening at the site of the fracture.

What can be done to correct a poor result after the setting of a fracture of the nose?

Plastic surgery can be performed to restore the nose to normal appearance.

DEVIATED SEPTUM

What is a deviated nasal septum?

The nasal septum is the partition in the nose which divides it into two chambers. It is composed of cartilage and bone. When this partition is crooked and not in the midline, it is called a deviated or deflected septum.

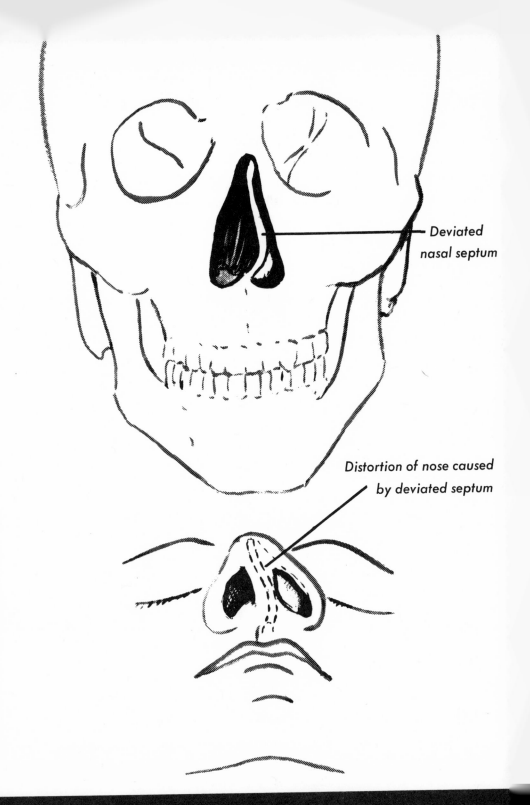

Deviated nasal septum

Distortion of nose caused by deviated septum

Deviated Nasal Septum. This is a common condition affecting the nose. It may occur as a result of injury or it may be present from birth. A markedly deviated septum interferes with normal breathing and should be corrected surgically.

What causes a septum to become deviated?

Many cases are due to faulty development. However, injuries to the nose, such as dislocation or fracture, can cause the formation of this defect.

Does the presence of a deviated septum cause symptoms?

Usually not. Many people have markedly deflected septums without nasal blockage. When there are symptoms, it takes the form of blockage of the free and easy passage of air through one nostril.

How can a deviated septum which causes nasal blockage be corrected?

This is corrected by performing an operation known as submucous resection of the nasal septum.

Is a submucous resection a dangerous operation?

No. The operation is performed through an intranasal incision. The membranes on either side of the bony and cartilaginous septum are elevated, and spurs, ridges, and deformed sections of the bone and cartilage are cut away. The operation is performed under local anesthesia.

At what age should submucous resection be carried out?

As this is an elective operation, it should not be done until the nasal bones have developed full growth, usually when the patient is about seventeen years of age.

How successful are operations for deviated septum?

In well-selected cases, the results are exceptionally good.

Are there any complications to this operation?

Very rarely, there may be bleeding when the nasal packing is removed. This can be readily controlled by the surgeon.

How soon after an operation for a deviated septum can one return to work?

Usually within ten to fourteen days.

How long a period of hospitalization is necessary?

One to two days.

NASAL POLYPS

What are nasal polyps?

They are grapelike masses of swollen tissue which protrude from the sinuses and the side walls of the nose.

What are thought to be the causes of nasal polyps?

They are thought to be due to an allergy.

What symptoms are caused by nasal polyps?

If the polyps are small and few in number, there may be no symptoms. Frequently, they will be large enough to obstruct the airway and cause difficulty in breathing. Occasionally, polyps will be so large as to extrude from the nostrils.

What is the treatment for nasal polyps?

When polyps are obstructive, they should be removed surgically. However, the basic treatment should be directed toward determining the cause of the condition and toward preventing recurrence of the polyps.

What operation is performed for the removal of the polyps?

A polypectomy is usually performed under local anesthesia in the surgeon's office or in the hospital. The polyps are grasped with a wire snare and removed as close to their attachment as possible.

Does this operation keep one from work for a long time?

No. Most patients may return to work the day following surgery.

NASAL SINUSES

What are the nasal sinuses, and where are they located?

The sinuses are mucous-membrane-lined air spaces, and are located

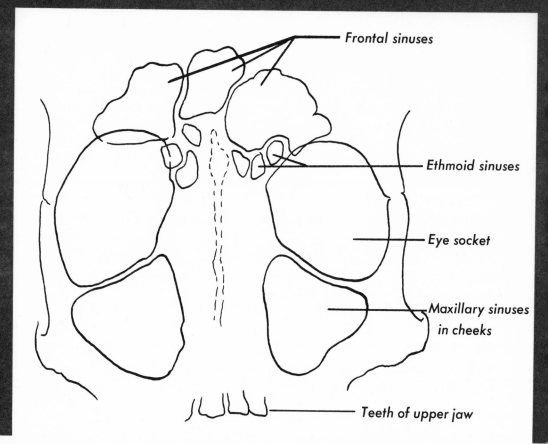

Frontal sinuses

Ethmoid sinuses

Eye socket

Maxillary sinuses
in cheeks

Teeth of upper jaw

Diagram of the Nasal Sinuses. Sinuses are air spaces within the bones of the skull whose main purposes are to lighten the skull and to give resonance to the voice. The sinuses are a frequent site of infection and, unfortunately, these infections tend to be chronic.

within the bones of the face and skull. They communicate, through small openings, with the nasal cavity. The frontal sinuses are located within the bone just above and behind the eyebrows; the maxillary sinuses are located within the bones of the cheeks beneath the eyes; the ethmoid sinuses are located near the side of the nose and inner aspect of the eyes and extend backward into the skull; and the sphenoid sinus is located deep in the skull above the level of the throat.

What is the function of the sinuses?

These air-lined spaces lighten the weight of the head and contribute toward the resonance of the voice.

Is inflammation of the sinuses (sinusitis) a common condition?

Sinusitis is one of the most common conditions encountered in the entire field of medicine. It consists of an inflammation of the mucous-membrane lining of one or more of the sinuses. When all the sinuses are involved, the condition is called pansinusitis.

What causes sinusitis?

It is usually secondary to an infection in the nasal cavity, although the maxillary sinus may become infected as a result of an extension from a tooth infection in the upper jaw. Swimming, diving, and injuries or fractures of the bones overlying the sinuses may also cause inflammation to take place. Anatomical deformities which block the sinus openings and allergies with nasal polyp formation may also predispose to sinusitis.

What are the symptoms of sinusitis?

They vary according to the sinus involved. The most common symptoms are:

a. Tenderness over the infected sinus.

b. A nasal quality to the voice.

c. Nasal obstruction, with discharge from the nose.

d. Severe headache, worse on lowering the head.

e. Elevated temperature.

How is the diagnosis of sinusitis made?

Sinusitis is usually suspected when a cold has persisted for more than one week. The presence of pain or tenderness over the affected sinus, headache, and the symptoms enumerated above will tend to establish the diagnosis. It can be confirmed by transillumination of the sinus with a strong light in a dark room and by taking x-rays.

Which sinuses are most prone to develop inflammation?

The maxillary, frontal, and ethmoid sinuses.

What is the treatment for sinusitis?

Most cases will respond well to medical treatment. This should consist of bed rest, steam inhalations, warm compresses to the affected

949

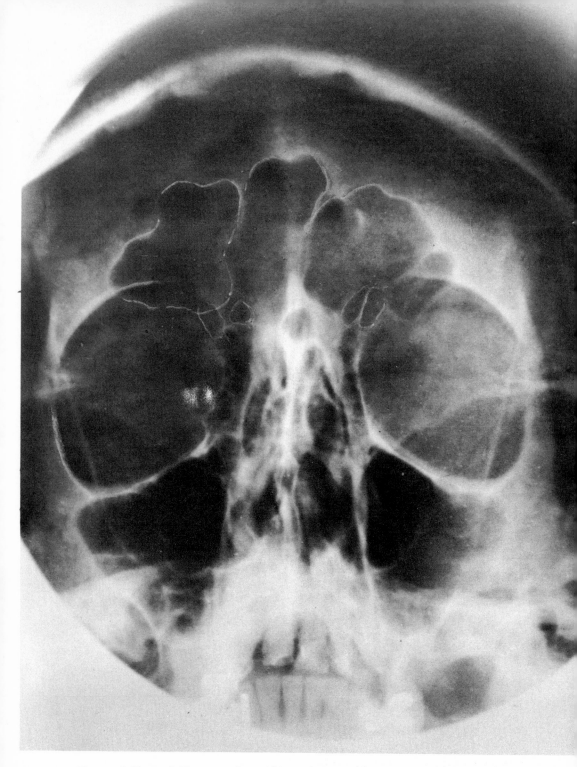

X-ray of Normal Sinuses. Pus within a sinus would appear as a haze on the x-ray film. Modern methods of treating sinus infections—especially the antibiotic drugs—have greatly improved the chances for cure.

sinus area, nose drops to lessen the congestion of the nasal mucous membranes, and the use of antibiotic and antihistaminic drugs. If the fever is high, medicines such as aspirin should be used. If the pain is severe, pain-relieving drugs such as codeine may be used. Further medical treatment in the physician's office will consist of nasal packs and various methods of removing the nasal discharge by the use of suction..Cultures of the sinus discharge are frequently taken to determine the exact germ involved and to test the sensitivity of these bacteria to the various antibiotic drugs.

What cases of sinusitis require surgery?

Those that fail, after a prolonged period of time, to respond to the above-mentioned medical management.

What operations are carried out for sinusitis?

The aim of all operations for sinusitis is to obtain adequate drainage and, in some cases, to remove diseased mucous membranes and bone. Most of these operations are done under local anesthesia, but some may require general anesthesia.

What operations are usually performed upon the maxillary sinus?

a. Simple puncture of the sinus through the nose, with irrigation and suction.

b. The cutting of a large window in the side wall of the nose into the sinus to promote drainage.

c. A radical sinusotomy, in which the mucous membrane lining the sinus is lifted away from the underlying bone and scraped out. In this operation, the incision is made inside the mouth beneath the upper lip.

What operations are performed on the frontal sinus?

Formerly, the frontal sinus was irrigated through the nose, but this is done rarely today. If surgery is necessary, an incision is made in the skin below the inner portion of the eyebrow and a small hole is cut in the bony floor of the frontal sinus. If the infection has involved the surrounding bone, it may become necessary to do a radical frontal sinusotomy. In this event, a larger incision is made and the entire bony floor of the frontal sinus is removed with a chisel. Al-

951

though frontal sinus operations are serious, the results are usually good and the majority of patients recover completely.

What operations are performed on the ethmoid sinuses?

These sinuses can usually be approached and scraped out through the nose. If the infection is severe or has involved the sphenoid sinus or has broken through to involve the tissues about the eyes, it may be necessary to do an external ethmoidectomy. In this event, the incision is simply a prolongation downward of the same type of incision that is made for a frontal sinus infection.

What operations are used for inflammation of the sphenoid sinus?

Under local anesthesia, this sinus can be probed and irrigated through the nose. As a severe sphenoid infection may lead to brain infection or blindness, it is sometimes necessary to do a radical operation in conjunction with a complete ethmoidectomy.

How effective is sinus surgery?

The great majority of cases are improved through surgery.

How long a hospital stay is necessary after major sinus surgery?

Usually seven to ten days.

Does sinusitis ever recur after surgery?

Yes, but in a small minority of cases.

How does one treat recurrent sinusitis?

It is treated as a new infection and is handled in the same way as an original infection.

TUMORS OF THE NOSE AND SINUSES

Are tumors of the nose and sinuses common?

The benign tumors are rather common. Among these, one would include nasal polyps, warts, and hemangiomas (small blood vessel tumors). Fortunately, malignant tumors are not very common in this area.

What is the treatment for benign tumors of the nose or sinuses?

Most of these can be removed readily under local anesthesia in the surgeon's office.

What is the treatment for malignant tumors of the nose and sinuses?

Cancer of the nose or sinuses is treated by wide surgical removal of the growth and surrounding tissues. Extensive plastic surgery is usually performed at a later date, after the physician is reasonably sure that all of the cancer was completely removed.

How successful is surgery for tumors of the nose and sinuses?

Surgery for benign tumors is uniformly successful. The success of surgery for cancer depends upon the time at which the surgery is performed and upon the degree of malignancy. If the surgery has been done before the cancer has spread to distant tissues, the expectation of cure is good. Modern surgical techniques may include the lifesaving measures in which large sections of the nose, face, cheek, the roof of the mouth, or the floor of the eye are removed.

Can cosmetic reconstruction be carried out after radical surgery upon the nose and sinuses?

Yes. Modern advances in technique in plastic surgery can effect remarkable restoration toward normal appearance.

NOSEBLEEDS

What causes nosebleeds?

There may be local or general causes or a combination of both. In many cases, there is no apparent cause.

What are some of the local causes of nosebleed?

  a. Injury to the nose or the base of the skull, with or without fracture.
  b. Foreign body in the nose.
  c. Operations upon the nose.
  d. Violent coughing, sneezing, or noseblowing.

e. Nose picking.

f. Ulcerations caused by disease, such as syphilis and tuberculosis.

g. Benign or malignant tumors within the nose or sinuses.

h. Varicose veins of the mucous membranes of the nose.

i. An acute inflammation of the mucous membrane lining of the nose, as occurs in allergy, sinusitis, or the common cold.

What are some of the general causes of nosebleeds?

a. High blood pressure.

b. Blood disorders, such as hemophilia, pernicious anemia, purpura, scurvy, leukemia, and jaundice.

c. Atmospheric changes, such as mountain climbing, diving, or descending to great depths within the sea.

How can one distinguish between a nosebleed caused by a local condition and one caused by a general condition?

If the bleeding arises from one nostril only, the cause is more likely to be local. Also, thorough nasal examination will reveal a bleeding point or other local cause.

How can nosebleeds be controlled?

There are really two types of nosebleeds. Over 90 per cent occur in the anterior part of the nose, arising from the septum or more rarely from the anterior ethmoid area. The point of bleeding can usually be found and controlled by cauterization under local anesthesia. This can be done by chemicals such as silver nitrate or chromic acid, or by electric coagulation.

What should be done as a first-aid measure for nosebleed?

Since the vast majority occur in the anterior part of the nasal septum, they can be controlled by simple continuous pressure applied to the side of the nose from which the bleeding arises. It is well to put a small piece of cotton in the nose, possibly moistened with some nose drop, if available. Pressure against this piece of cotton should be maintained for at least ten minutes. The person should be sitting up, with his head tilted forward, to prevent blood from trickling down his throat.

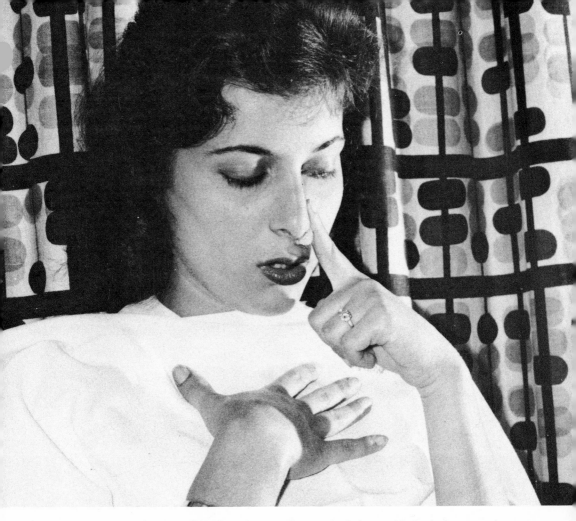

Packing the Nose for Nosebleed. The nostril is packed thoroughly with cotton and the head is bent forward slightly. The index finger is then pressed firmly against the side of the nose in which the cotton has been placed and is held there for several minutes. This procedure will control most nosebleeds.

What can be done for bleeding arising from the posterior part of the nose?

This type cannot be self-treated. People with this condition must be hospitalized, as it is usually necessary to pack the posterior part of the nose through the mouth.

How long is the nasal packing left in place?

The posterior packing is left in place for about one week. Anterior packing should be removed gradually, starting generally about the fourth day.

What is the treatment for nosebleeds which arise from a general condition?

Expert medical advice must be obtained and treatment of the underlying disease must be instituted.

PLASTIC SURGERY OF THE NOSE
(*Rhinoplasty*)

Can all nasal deformities be corrected through plastic surgery?

Almost every deformity can be corrected to a certain degree.

What are the common types of nasal deformity?

a. A twisted nose.

b. Deformities of the tip of the nose or nostrils.

c. Depression of the bridge and ridge of the nose, called "saddle nose."

d. Hump nose or hook nose.

Is there a standard appearance for the nose?

No. Different peoples and races have different standards of beauty or acceptability. However, in today's society the most acceptable and pleasing angle between the lip and the nose is an angle of between ninety and ninety-five degrees.

What is meant by the expression "a perfect nose"?

In the absolute sense, there is no such thing as a perfect nose. The best one can say is that a nose should fit the face.

What are some of the important factors in determining the results of plastic surgery upon the nose?

a. The age of the patient. The best results are obtained in those from sixteen to thirty years of age.

b. The skin. The quality of the skin, including its thickness, thinness, and tendency toward oiliness.

c. The extent of the deformity. The greater the deformity, the more difficult it is to get a perfect result.

d. The type of deformity. Certain types of deformity are much harder to cure than others.

e. The mental stability of the patient. The results are poorer among neurotic patients who have a tendency to worry about insignificant defects.

Are the results good when an operation is performed upon a child rather than upon an adult?

The surgeon should wait until the nose is fully formed; this does not take place until the child has attained at least the age of sixteen.

What operation is performed for a plastic procedure on the nose?

All the incisions are made within the nose and the skin of the nose is loosened or undermined to free it from the bone and cartilage that make up the framework of the nose. The framework of the nose is then cut and shaped according to a plan laid out before operation. The skin then falls back upon the reshaped framework and is sutured into position. Packing is placed within the nose and a dressing is placed on the outside of the nose to help maintain the new position of the bone and cartilage. As time passes, the skin will attach itself to the newly shaped bony and cartilaginous framework of the nose.

Are any scars visible after plastic operations upon the nose?

No.

Is it possible for the patient to select the type of nose he desires?

Only to a certain degree. The surgeon must first overcome the defects of the nose and then he will try to create a result pleasing to his patient. The patient must understand clearly before surgery that an exact prediction cannot be made as to the specific appearance of the nose after surgery.

Can the patient obtain a good approximate idea of what his nose will look like after surgery?

Yes. An approximation can be foretold.

What materials are used to build up a nose?

The best substance or graft is a piece of bone or cartilage taken from

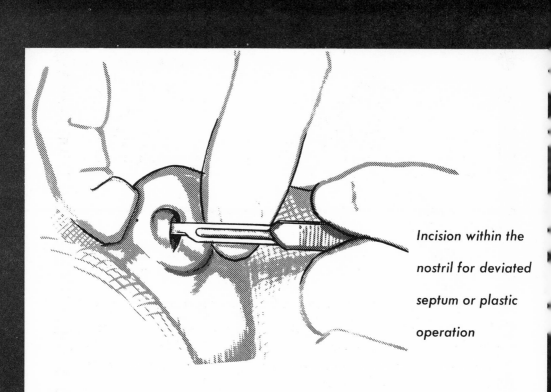

Incision within the nostril for deviated septum or plastic operation

Incision within the nostril for shortening of the septum during plastic operation

Plastic Surgery upon the Nose. The incisions for plastic operations upon the nose are made within the nostril so that no scar will be visible after the operation is completed. Considerable swelling follows most nasal plastic operations and it may take several weeks or months for it to subside completely.

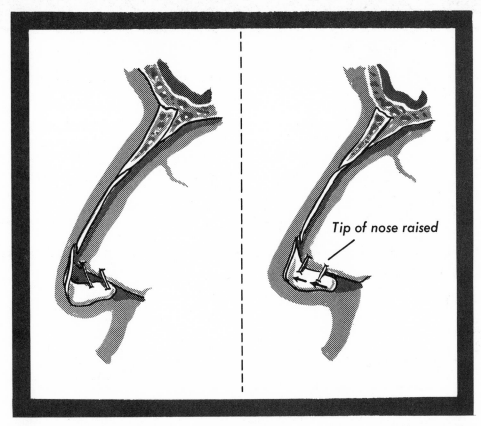

Plastic Surgery upon the Nose. Plastic operations on the nose are usually performed under local anesthesia and require but a short hospital stay. Although marked improvement follows almost all plastic operations upon the nose, the patient should understand that the exact shape the nose will take cannot always be predicted.

the patient himself. This is usually taken from the hip bone or from a rib cartilage.

How long does a plastic operation on the nose take to perform?

Approximately one hour.

What anesthesia is used?

Local anesthesia, fortified by sedation.

Are plastic operations upon the nose painful procedures?

No.

How long a hospital stay is necessary?

Two to four days.

Is it common for the eyes to be discolored or swollen after this operation?

Yes. This will begin to subside in approximately forty-eight hours, but may not completely disappear for a week or two.

When are the dressings and packings removed from the nose after a plastic operation?

In five to seven days.

How long after a plastic operation on the nose can one breathe normally?

After removal of the intranasal packing, about the fifth to seventh day.

Does a plastic operation upon the nose affect the sense of smell?

No.

After a nose has healed completely following a plastic operation, must special care be exercised not to injure it?

No. A healed nose following plastic surgery is just as strong as any other nose.

Do noses which have undergone plastic surgery tend to sag and change shape months or years later?

No. They will heal in the position which is present immediately following the surgical procedure.

May swelling of the nose persist even for several months after plastic surgery?

Yes. It may take several months or even a year for the nose to attain its absolute permanent shape and for *all* of the swelling to disappear.

How soon after a plastic operation on the nose can one return to work and to social functions?

In approximately two weeks, even though some swelling may remain.

Is it possible to repeat a plastic operation if the result of the first operation is unsatisfactory?

Yes; but it is best to wait several months before repeating the surgery, so that stabilization of healing has had an opportunity to develop.

How successful are plastic operations upon the nose?

The over-all improvement is almost always good and the general degree of satisfaction is high. When results are poor, they can often be remedied by reoperation.

 *The Pancreas*

Where is the pancreas, and what are its functions?

The pancreas is a flat yellowish gland which stretches across the upper abdomen for a distance of approximately five inches. It lies on the posterior abdominal wall, between the lowermost extent of the stomach and the upper margin of the transverse colon. Its head is attached to, and is surrounded by, the curve of the duodenum. The pancreas has two main functions:

a. To manufacture various enzymes (chemical substances) which help to digest the food in the intestinal tract.

b. To manufacture and secrete into the bloodstream the hormone known as insulin, which regulates the rate at which sugar is utilized by the body.

How do pancreatic secretions reach the intestines?

Through long ducts or tubes which course the entire width of the pancreas and empty into the duodenum.

How does an upset in the pancreas become evident?

There may be upper abdominal pain, with nausea and vomiting, particularly after eating large meals. Failure to produce sufficient insulin will become evident by the development of diabetes.

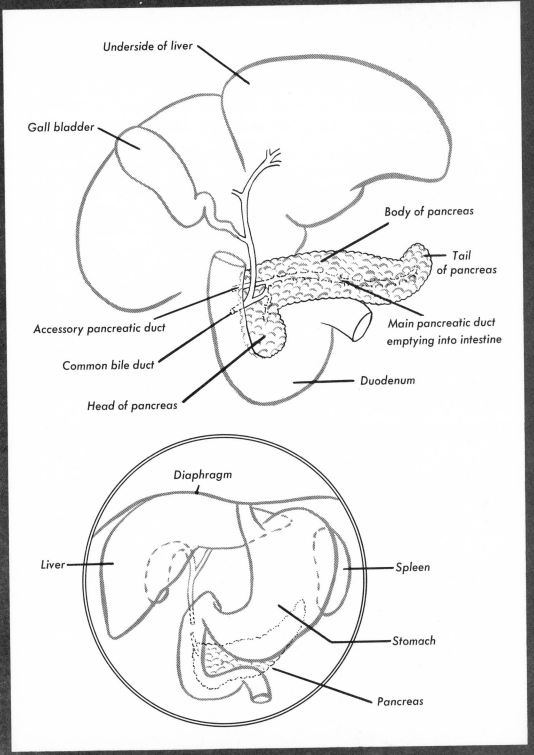

Anatomy of the Pancreas. This diagram shows the location and the relations of the pancreatic gland within the upper portion of the abdomen. The pancreas is important in that it secretes enzymes which help to digest food. It is also the organ which manufactures insulin, the hormone which controls the metabolism of sugar. Failure of the insulin-producing cells within the pancreas results in diabetes.

What are the most common diseases of the pancreas?

a. Pancreatitis.

1. The acute type. 2. The chronic or recurring type.

b. Abscess of the pancreas.

c. Diabetes. (See Chapter 18, on Diabetes.)

d. Hyperinsulinism, or overproduction of the hormone which causes sugar to be burned by the body.

e. Cysts of the pancreas.

f. Benign tumors of the pancreas.

g. Cancer of the pancreas.

PANCREATITIS
(Inflammation of the Pancreas)

What causes acute inflammations of the pancreas (pancreatitis)?

In some instances, it is thought to be caused by infected bile backing up into the pancreatic ducts; in other instances, it is caused by bacteria which invade the pancreas directly through its blood supply. It is not unusual for pancreatitis to have its onset shortly after one has eaten large quantities of food or imbibed excessive amounts of alcohol.

Is pancreatitis a serious disease?

Yes, especially in its acute form, which can be accompanied by severe hemorrhage, overwhelming toxemia, and death. However, serious as it is, the great majority of those affected will recover.

What are the symptoms and signs of acute pancreatitis?

a. Elevation of temperature.

b. Pain, tenderness, and distention in the upper abdomen.

c. Nausea and vomiting.

d. An increase in the quantity of amylase and lipase (chemical enzymes) circulating in the blood.

e. Signs of shock in severe cases, secondary to hemorrhage and toxemia.

What are the symptoms of chronic or recurring pancreatitis?

When it recurs, it usually takes the form of an acute episode. Chronic indigestion, a bloated feeling, and vague abdominal pains are seen in the chronic form of the disease.

What is the treatment for acute pancreatitis?

a. No food by mouth is given; fluids and glucose (sugar) are given through the veins.

b. Atropine, banthine, or similar drugs are administered to inhibit pancreatic activity.

c. Antibiotics are sometimes given to control bacterial infection within the gland.

Is a patient with acute pancreatitis often subjected to surgery?

Yes. Surgery is often recommended because the exact diagnosis has not been established and it is necessary to rule out other upper abdominal emergencies for which surgery is mandatory. Surgery is also performed for the complications of pancreatitis, such as abscess or cyst formation.

What operative procedures are carried out when operating upon pancreatitis?

The fluid which is secreted into the abdominal cavity in cases of pancreatitis is drained. If the gall bladder or bile ducts are found to contain stones and if it is thought that this is a contributing factor in the causation of the pancreatitis, the stones are removed and the gall bladder or bile ducts are drained with rubber tubes.

Does disease within the gall bladder or biliary system often incite pancreatitis?

Approximately half the cases of pancreatitis are associated with gallstones, and many physicians feel that this is one of the main factors leading to the development of pancreatitis.

Does pancreatitis have a tendency to recur?

Yes, unless the underlying condition, such as gall bladder disease, is corrected.

965

How can pancreatitis best be prevented?

By eating a bland low-fat diet. By not overeating, and by restricting alcohol intake. Also, any disease within the gall bladder or bile ducts must be eradicated.

Is pancreatitis usually associated with diabetes?

Usually not. It is remarkable that those cells that manufacture insulin do not appear to be involved very often when pancreatitis occurs. It is only in the very severe case that diabetes may ensue.

ABSCESS OF THE PANCREAS

When is an abscess of the pancreas most apt to develop?

Following an attack of acute pancreatitis.

Does this occur frequently?

No. It is found usually only after very severe cases, where the pancreatitis has caused destruction of a portion of the gland.

How is a diagnosis of pancreatic abscess made?

By studying the history of a previous episode of pancreatitis, and by noting pain and tenderness in the upper abdomen, along with temperature elevation. These symptoms come on several days or weeks after an attack of pancreatitis has appeared to subside.

What is the treatment for an abscess within the pancreas?

  a. Administration of antibiotic drugs.
  b. Surgical drainage of the abscess.

What are the chances for recovery following surgery for a pancreatic abscess?

The great majority of patients will get well, but the wound may drain pus for quite some time.

DIABETES
(See Chapter 18, on Diabetes.)

HYPERINSULINISM

What is hyperinsulinism?

It is a condition in which the insulin-producing cells (the cells of the Islets of Langerhans) manufacture and secrete an excessive amount of insulin into the bloodstream.

What causes hyperinsulinism?

Some cases are caused by a tumor (adenoma) within the pancreas involving an overgrowth of those cells which manufacture insulin. Other cases are caused by an upset in metabolism of the gland, with resultant secretion of abnormally large quantities of insulin into the bloodstream.

What are the symptoms of hyperinsulinism?

Abrupt episodes of intense hunger, trembling of the hands, black spots before the eyes, mental confusion, fainting, and, in severe cases, convulsions with loss of consciousness. Examination of the blood at the time of these attacks will show an extremely low level of circulating sugar.

What type of person is most likely to be affected by hyperinsulinism?

Young adults are more prone than older people to develop hyperinsulinism.

Is hyperinsulinism always accompanied by a tumor of the pancreas?

No. There are many cases in which examination of the pancreas will reveal no abnormality. Microscopic examination of a portion of the pancreas, however, may sometimes show overgrowth of the insulin-producing cells without true tumor formation.

How large are adenomas of the pancreas?

They are small lesions measuring no more than one-half to one inch in diameter. They cannot be felt on abdominal examination.

What is the treatment for hyperinsulinism?

At first, medical management is attempted. This will consist largely of giving low quantities of sugar in the diet so as not to excite or

overstimulate insulin production. If this form of treatment is unsuccessful, then an exploratory abdominal operation is carried out for
the presence of a tumor (pancreatic adenoma).

What form of surgery is carried out for hyperinsulinism when no tumor of the pancreas is discovered at operation?

Some surgeons feel that a portion, such as a third or a half, of the
pancreas should be removed. Others feel that this is not beneficial
and carries with it too great a risk.

If a benign adenoma of the pancreas is found, can it be removed surgically?

Yes. This is not a dangerous procedure and the patient is usually
cured of his hyperinsulinism.

Does recovery from hyperinsulinism take place?

Yes, in the great majority of cases. However, it is important to carry
out a thorough examination of the patient to make sure that some
other endocrine gland, such as the pituitary, thyroid, or adrenal, is
not responsible for the upset in pancreatic function.

CYSTS OF THE PANCREAS

What are cysts of the pancreas, and how often do they occur?

It is thought that blockage of one of the pancreatic ducts may cause
cysts to form, or that they are the end result of an episode of pancreatitis. When cysts do occur (they are an uncommon lesion), they
may vary in size from that of a grape to a watermelon.

Are cysts of the pancreas dangerous?

No. The small ones may be ignored. It is only the large ones that
require attention when they press upon and interfere with the function of neighboring organs.

How is the diagnosis of a cyst of the pancreas arrived at?

The larger cysts can be felt by the examining physician as a painless,
rounded swelling in the upper abdomen.

What surgery is advocated for a cyst of the pancreas?

The cyst is removed or, if this is not technically feasible because of its size, attachments, or location, it is merely drained of its fluid contents. Several rubber drains are inserted into the cyst cavity and are left in place for several weeks, until the cyst collapses and fills in by itself. In some cases, the wall of the cyst is stitched to the stomach and its contents permitted to drain internally. This method often leads to a rapid cure.

Are there any permanent after-effects from cysts of the pancreas?

No. Digestion and pancreatic function usually return to normal within several weeks to a few months.

BENIGN TUMORS OF THE PANCREAS

What is the most common benign tumor of the pancreas?

A growth involving those cells that manufacture insulin. (See the section on Hyperinsulinism in this chapter.)

Do these benign tumors ever develop into cancer?

Yes. This is one of the main reasons why surgery should be undertaken when a pancreatic tumor is suspected.

CANCER OF THE PANCREAS

Is cancer of the pancreas encountered very often?

Unfortunately, it is one of the most common of all abdominal cancers and carries with it the lowest rate of permanent cure.

What causes cancer of the pancreas?

The cause is not known.

Where are most cancers of the pancreas located?

The majority are located in the head of the pancreas, adjoining the duodenum. Most benign tumors of this organ are located further to the left side in the body or tail of the pancreas.

What are symptoms of cancer of the pancreas?

Pain in the upper abdomen, usually radiating to the back. Also, because the cancer is usually located in the head of the pancreas, its growth creates pressure on the bile ducts and this will result in obstruction and the slow onset of jaundice. The patient experiences loss of appetite, weight loss, and progressive weakness.

What are the chances for cure in cancer of the pancreas?

Not very great, although operations have been evolved in which the entire pancreas and the surrounding duodenum can be removed. Unfortunately, even with these extensive procedures, it is not often that the cancer can be eradicated completely.

Will the patient develop diabetes after removal of the pancreas?

Yes. However, other organs in the body tend to take over the metabolism of sugar and the patient often does not die from diabetes.

What is the life expectancy after a diagnosis of cancer of the pancreas has been made?

Approximately six to eighteen months. It must be remembered, though, that isolated cases have been reported in which permanent cure has followed removal of the entire gland.

Parasites and Parasitic Diseases

CHAPTER 46

What is an animal parasite?

One which lives at the expense of its host.

Are there organisms other than animal which are parasitic?

Yes. Parasites include bacteria, viruses, and fungi, as well as animals. However, in the medical sense, parasitology (the study of parasites) is generally restricted to the animal parasites of man.

How do parasites gain entry to the human body?

Through contaminated food or drink, by direct contact with the skin or mucous membranes, or through infected blood-sucking insects.

What are common parasites which gain entry to the body by means of contaminated food or drink?

These include intestinal protozoa (endamoeba histolytica and balantidium coli), roundworms (ascaris lumbricoides and enterobius vermicularis), tapeworms such as the fish tapeworm (diphyllobothrium latum) or the beef tapeworm (taenia solium), etc.

What are examples of parasites which gain entrance through the skin or mucous membranes?

Hookworms, and the itch mite.

What is the most common parasite to be transmitted by an infected blood-sucking insect?

The malarial parasite, which is transmitted by an infected mosquito.

Once parasites gain access to the body, can they multiply there?

Not all animal parasites multiply in the body. This is particularly true of infestations with worms. However, the malarial parasites and amoebae, among others, multiply within the body.

Is anyone actually immune to parasitic infestation?

No.

How can parasitic disease be avoided?

The practice of good sanitary habits, having a pure water supply, avoidance of contact with infected material, and control of carriers of infection (mosquitoes, lice, etc.) are some of the best means of avoiding infection. Some of these involve measures of public health that may be world-wide in scope, such as the control of mosquitoes, ticks, etc.

Is it possible to harbor more than one parasite at a time?

Yes. Multiple infestation is very common.

Are there any areas of the world where parasitic diseases are more prevalent than others?

Yes. People living in the tropics or semi-tropics have a relatively high incidence of parasitic infestation. Those areas where sanitation is poorly handled also have a high incidence of parasitism. Food habits are also important. Scandinavians who commonly eat or sample raw fish have higher infection rates from the fish tapeworm than people who are careful to cook this food thoroughly before eating.

How is a diagnosis of parasitic disease made?

The only certain way is by identifying the organism in body excrement (stool or urine), body fluids, or tissues. At times, skin testing and other laboratory tests may be helpful in arriving at a precise diagnosis.

Are there any specific blood changes in parasitic disease?

No, although an increase in the number of certain circulating white blood cells (eosinophils) may be suggestive. In malaria, or certain other parasitic diseases, the parasite may be identified microscopically by examining a blood smear. In such cases, an absolute diagnosis can be made.

Is there any effective treatment to cure parasitic diseases?

In most instances, specific treatment *is* available and the infestation can be eradicated. The treatment, however, varies with each particular parasite.

AMEBIASIS

What is amebiasis?

This is an infection from a one-celled animal parasite, called an amoeba. There are several types of amoebae which are disease producing, the most important of which is called endamoeba histolytica. It generally causes an intestinal disease known as amoebic colitis, or dysentery. The parasite may at times invade other organs of the body, including the liver and brain.

Where is amebiasis found?

It is found throughout the world, but most commonly in the tropics and semi-tropics. It should be noted that there was quite an outbreak in the city of Chicago not too many years ago. With the vast increase in world travel, no country is immune to this type of infection.

How is amebiasis transmitted?

From person to person through ingestion of food or drink contaminated with feces containing the cysts of this parasite.

What are the symptoms of amoebic colitis (dysentery)?

Recurrent attacks of diarrhea, abdominal pain, tenderness, and loss of weight.

973

How is the diagnosis made?

By demonstrating the parasite in the feces or tissues of the infected person.

Is amebiasis a serious disease?

Yes. Not only can debility be great, but severe infection may cause death. Furthermore, complications are not uncommon in untreated cases.

Are the chances for recovery favorable in amoebic dysentery?

Yes. There are several drugs which cure the great majority of cases. These include chiniofon, diodoquin, carbarsone, etc. Treatment must be intensive and should be supervised by an expert in the field.

Are there other protozoan parasites of the intestine?

Yes, but they are of minor importance.

TRICHOMONAS VAGINITIS

What is trichomonas vaginitis?

This is an infestation of the human vagina with the parasite trichomonas vaginalis. It can cause an inflammatory condition associated with a heavy vaginal discharge. Since the parasite is sometimes found in the male urethra, the infection can be readily passed from male to female.

Is trichomonas infection serious?

No. It is not a serious disease, but it sometimes proves difficult to eradicate completely. Recently, new fungicides taken orally, have proved most effective in overcoming these infestations.

LEISHMANIASIS

What is leishmaniasis?

It is a group of diseases caused by certain protozoan parasites called leishmania. These include kala azar, espundia, and oriental sore. These are serious diseases seen in tropical countries. Sometimes they are seen in the United States in returned military personnel who have served in infected areas. Kala azar has a very high mortality rate in untreated persons. Espundia and oriental sore are diseases in which the skin is principally affected. The outlook in these conditions is much better than in kala azar and treatment is usually curative.

AFRICAN SLEEPING SICKNESS

What is African sleeping sickness?

This is a parasitic disease caused by a protozoan called trypanosoma. There are at least two different types known. The disease is transmitted by biting flies (tsetse flies). The disease is extremely serious and, unless treated, death occurs in most cases.

CHAGAS' DISEASE

What is Chagas' disease?

This is a disease caused by a trypanosoma which is limited to the Western Hemisphere, notably to Brazil. It is transmitted by the bite of a triatomid bug. The disease is a serious one and is attended with a high mortality rate.

MALARIA

What are the various types of malaria?

There are at least three different types, each caused by a different malarial parasite. These include tertian malaria caused by plasmodium vivax, quartan malaria caused by plasmodium malariae, and estivo-autumnal malaria caused by plasmodium falciparum.

How is malaria transmitted to man?

By inoculation through the bite of an infected anopheles mosquito.

Where do the malaria parasites live in man?

In the red blood cells, which they destroy.

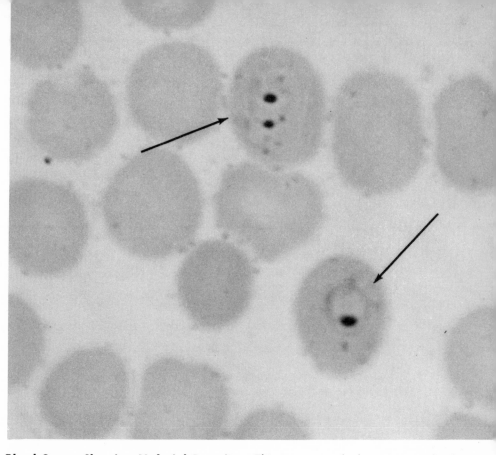

Blood Smear Showing Malarial Parasite. This is an actual photomicrograph of a blood smear showing malarial parasites within the red blood cell. Although malaria is still one of the most prevalent diseases in the world, it has been eradicated from most civilized countries by extensive mosquito-control programs.

How are the different types of malarial parasites distinguished?

By their specific appearance in the blood and by the difference in clinical picture and symptoms which each produces.

Where is malaria found?

It is undoubtedly one of the most important diseases of the warm climates of the world. However, it is found as far north as southern Sweden.

Are any people immune to malaria?

All native races where malaria is common have a considerable resistance to the disease, but this may be the result of repeated infections causing a build-up of relative resistance. In all probability, there is little or no natural immunity to malaria.

What are the symptoms of malaria?

Episodes of shaking chills and fever, in severe paroxysms, usually spaced at regular intervals.

What is the outlook for untreated malaria?

Untreated malaria is rarely fatal except in the estivo-autumnal type, where the outlook is always grave.

What is the treatment for malaria?

There are a number of drugs which are very effective against the malarial parasites. These include chloroquine, quinine and plasmochin.

Can these drugs be used successfully to suppress or prevent the development of malaria?

Yes.

Should an individual known to have had malaria ever be used as a blood donor?

No. Such an individual might be a carrier of the parasites, and the disease could thereby be transmitted to the recipient of the blood transfusion.

WORM DISEASES

What are roundworms?

Roundworms are animals that vary in size from forms barely visible to the naked eye to those which are as large around as a lead pencil and almost a foot in length. They look something like an ordinary earthworm.

What are some of the roundworms which infest man?

These include trichinella spiralis (trichinosis); ascaris lumbricoides (common roundworm of hogs and man); necator americanus (North American hookworm); ancylostoma duodenale (Old World hookworm); etc.

How is trichinosis acquired?

The parasites normally form cysts in the muscles of hogs. When pork that is incompletely cooked is eaten by man, the parasites are released in the body and make their way into the muscles of man.

Is trichinosis a common disease?

Yes. It has been estimated that almost twenty-eight million persons throughout the world are infested, three-fourths of whom live in North America.

Is trichinosis a serious disease?

Although trichinosis is rarely fatal, a serious infection can cause death.

Can trichinosis be treated successfully?

Once the parasites enter the muscles, there is no specific treatment.

Can trichinosis be prevented?

Yes, by thoroughly cooking pork and pork products before eating.

Where does the human whipworm reside?

The whipworm (trichuris trichiura) normally resides in the cecum and appendix of man.

How is whipworm infection acquired?

By eating the eggs of the whipworm, which reside in soil contaminated by feces.

How is the diagnosis of whipworm infection made?

By finding the eggs in the human stool.

Can whipworms cause appendicitis?

Occasionally, the worms may provoke an attack of acute appendicitis, but this is not held to be one of the truly frequent causes.

How can infection be prevented?

Sanitary disposal of feces and thorough washing of the hands before meals are effective preventive measures.

How do hookworms get into the human body?

Free-living larval forms can penetrate the intact skin. They generally gain access through the skin between the toes of individuals who walk barefoot in soil contaminated with human feces.

Is hookworm infection a serious disease?

Yes. The disease is extremely common in the Southern states, where it causes severe anemia, malnutrition, and diarrhea. "Potbelly" is a common finding in children infected with hookworm disease.

What is "ground itch"?

This is the first lesion produced by hookworms as they gain access to the body through the skin.

Where do the adult hookworms reside?

In the intestinal canal.

How is the diagnosis of hookworm made?

By finding the eggs in the human stool.

How can hookworm disease be prevented?

As in most roundworm diseases, it is important to dispose of human feces carefully. Also, in infected areas, it is most important to wear shoes at all times!

Where does the human pinworm, or seatworm, normally reside?

In the cecum, appendix, and large intestine.

Why are they called seatworms?

Because they tend to migrate about the anus, especially at night, and cause severe itching in that region of the body.

What types of individuals are most commonly infected with pinworms?

Children.

Do pinworms ever infect an entire family?

Yes. This is common.

How does one get a pinworm infection?

By eating the eggs of pinworms. Scratching the infected skin about the anal area may result in eggs being picked up by the fingernails. If the hands and nails are then not cleaned frequently and thoroughly, infection can be spread to others, or reinfection of the same individual can occur when the fingers are placed in the mouth.

How is a diagnosis of pinworm infection made?

By finding the eggs in the feces or perianal skin.

Do pinworms ever cause other diseases?

Yes. They are an occasional cause of acute appendicitis. Also, the severe itching they induce may result in nervousness, irritability, and emotional instability.

How can pinworm infection be prevented?

a. Scrupulous attention to personal hygiene is important.
b. The nails must be cut short.
c. Toilet seats must be thoroughly scrubbed.
d. Individuals known to be infected should be treated. Also, they must discontinue scratching themselves about the anal region.

Is the common roundworm of man (ascaris) the same as the one found in the intestine of hogs?

Apparently not. Although the two worms look exactly alike, infection from hog to man, or vice versa, does not occur.

Is ascaris infection very serious?

Usually not. Prompt treatment is curative.

What is filariasis?

This is a serious debilitating infection seen in the tropics, which is caused by a tiny worm (wuchereria bancrofti). The worms block the lymph channels of the limbs, resulting in tremendous enlargement of structures. The condition is also known as elephantiasis.

Is filariasis ever seen in this country?

Yes, but only in people who have returned from areas of the world where the disease is normally found.

What is a fluke worm?

This is a flatworm that has no true body cavity like the roundworms. The fluke worms generally have suckers, by means of which they attach themselves to the human body.

What fluke worms are parasitic in man?

The blood flukes or schistosomes, the Chinese liver fluke, the oriental lung fluke, and many others.

Where are the fluke worms found?

They are world-wide in distribution, but are mainly found in the warmer climates.

What are the common tapeworms infesting man?

a. The pork tapeworm (taenia solium).
b. The beef tapeworm (taenia saginata).
c. The fish tapeworm (diphyllobothrium latum).
d. The dog tapeworm (echinococcus granulosus).

Why are these worms called "tapeworms"?

Because they consist of a series of flat segments attached to a head (scolex) and because they resemble an elongated flat tape measure.

Where do tapeworms commonly reside?

In the intestine, where they anchor themselves by means of their scolex (head).

How is tapeworm infection usually acquired?

By eating foods which contain the larvae of the worms. Thus, the fish tapeworm is acquired by eating infected fish which has been improperly cooked, etc.

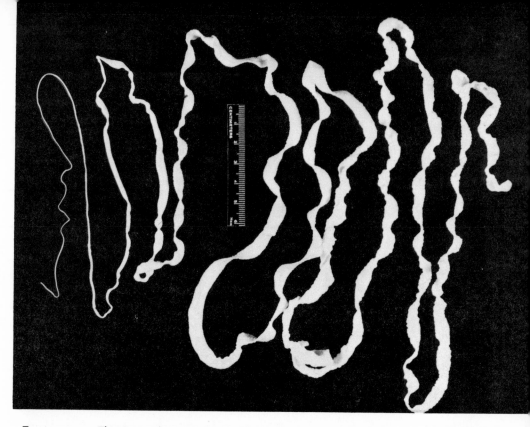

Tapeworm. This is a photograph of an actual tapeworm passed by the intestinal tract of a human being. Unless the head comes out with the tapeworm, it will continue to grow. There are many medications which will eliminate this parasite from the body.

How can tapeworm infection be prevented?

Proper cooking of fish, pork, or beef will kill the worms which they harbor. This will prevent infection from these parasites when the food is eaten.

In respect to other tapeworms, such as the dog tapeworm, care must be taken not to come in contact with the feces of these animals. Sanitary disposal of human and animal excretions is an important consideration.

How long do tapeworms measure?

They vary in length from a fraction of an inch, to over twenty feet for the beef tapeworm.

How is the diagnosis of tapeworm infection made?

When the adult worm inhabits the intestinal canal, the diagnosis is made by finding the eggs or segments of the worm in the feces.

Why is it necessary to recover the head or scolex of the worm in order to cure a tapeworm infection?

The worms grow from the head down. Unless the head is removed from the body, the worm will continue to live and grow.

How does one find the head?

In treated cases, the stool specimens are collected and carefully strained and examined for the presence of the scolex.

What is the treatment for the various types of intestinal worm infestations?

There are specific drugs which will kill the various worms which live in the human intestinal tract. Some of these medications, such as tetrachlorethylene and hexylresorcinol, can be used for several of the various types of worms. Other drugs, such as oil of chenopodium or gentian violet are more helpful in treating roundworms. It is important to seek medical advice for these conditions. When treated properly and intensively, most worm infections can be cured without leaving permanent ill effects.

What is an echinococcus cyst?

This is the larval form of the tapeworm of dogs, echinococcus granulosus. The adult worm is commonly infective of dogs. Man acts as the intermediate host. Commonly, sheep, cattle, and hogs are the reservoir hosts, but many cases of human infection are known.

Is an echinococcus infection serious in man?

Yes. The larvae invade the liver, lungs, and sometimes the brain, and may give rise to serious symptoms.

What is the treatment for an echinococcus infection in man?

It is generally surgical and will involve the removal of the cyst from the infected organ. This may be serious and dangerous if the brain, lung, or liver is involved.

47

The Parathyroid Glands

Where are the parathyroid glands, and what are their function?

They are four small, pea-sized structures located behind and attached to the thyroid gland in the neck. They are embedded within thyroid substance and are not easily located even when surgical dissection is carried out. The parathyroid glands secrete a hormone (parathormone) which is responsible for the maintenance of balance in calcium and phosphorous metabolism.

What happens when there is overproduction of parathyroid hormone (hyperparathyroidism)?

This results in an increase in the amount of calcium circulating in the bloodstream and in the excretion of an abnormally large amount of calcium in the urine.

What harm results from overactivity of the parathyroid glands?

a. It can lead to the formation of stones in the kidneys and subsequent impairment of kidney function.
b. Such overactivity can cause calcium to be withdrawn from the bones.

How is the diagnosis of parathyroid overactivity made?

By performing a blood chemical examination and finding a high level of calcium. Also, by noting characteristic changes in bony structure, as seen on x-ray examination.

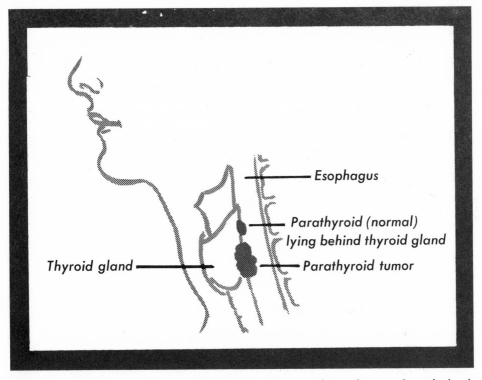

Esophagus

Parathyroid (normal)
lying behind thyroid gland

Thyroid gland

Parathyroid tumor

Anatomy of the Parathyroid Glands. This diagram shows the parathyroid glands as they are located behind the thyroid in the neck. One of these glands is pictured as normal in size; the larger one illustrates tumor formation. Parathyroid tumors, by stimulating excessive secretion of the parathyroid hormone, cause cyst formation and bone deformities. Surgical removal of a parathyroid tumor can be carried out successfully and will result in a cure.

What are the dangers of demineralization of calcium from the bones?

The bones become weakened, brittle, form cysts, and fracture easily.

Does overactivity of the parathyroid glands lead to marked bone deformity?

Yes. This condition, known as osteitis fibrosa cystica, is often associated with grotesque deformities of the bones.

What is the most common cause of overactivity of the parathyroid glands?

A tumor in one or more of the glands.

What is the treatment for hyperparathyroidism?

Surgical removal of the gland in which a tumor is present.

Is removal of a parathyroid tumor a dangerous operative procedure?

No. It is no more serious than an ordinary thyroid operation, and recovery can be anticipated without great disability or discomfort.

What type of incision is made in operating upon the parathyroid glands, and where on the body is the incision made?

The same type of collar incision across the lower neck as is made in performing a thyroid operation.

Are these scars disfiguring?

No. They usually heal as a thin white line.

Will the bone cysts heal and the bone deformities disappear after removal of a parathyroid tumor?

There is remarkable improvement after this procedure, in that the cysts fill in and calcium returns to the bone substance. However, all deformities do not disappear if they have been present for a long time or have been very extensive.

Is the cause for the hyperparathyroidism always found upon operation?

Not in all cases. Occasionally, despite all indications that a tumor is present, none is found in the neck. This may be due to the fact that a parathyroid gland has developed in an abnormal position in the neck, or even in the chest cavity. In such cases, to produce a cure, one must find the gland and remove it.

What symptoms are caused by underactivity of the parathyroid glands (hypoparathyroidism)?

a. Sudden spasms and cramps in various muscles.

b. In severe cases, tetany (convulsions) take place.

How is the diagnosis of underactivity of the parathyroids made?

a. By examining the blood and finding an abnormally low calcium level.

b. By tests which demonstrate excess muscle irritability.

c. By noting the occurrence of characteristic cramps of the muscles and tendons of the hands and feet, and by the onset of convulsive seizures (tetany).

What is the treatment for underactivity of the parathyroid glands?

a. Large doses of vitamin D, taken daily.

b. Large supplementary intake of calcium in the form of tablets.

Will this treatment cure underactivity of the parathyroids?

A cure will not result, but patients with this condition can be maintained in good health indefinitely by adequate doses of the above medications.

Is there any surgical treatment for underactivity of the parathyroids?

Attempts have been made to graft these glands from animals and humans, but most of these procedures have resulted in failure.

Is parathyroid function ever disturbed as a result of an operation upon the thyroid gland?

Yes. In complicated cases, usually those with recurrent goiter, the parathyroids are sometimes injured or inadvertently removed along with the goiter.

What happens when the parathyroid glands have all been removed?

Symptoms of underactivity (hypoparathyroidism), such as muscle cramps and tetany (convulsions), may develop.

Must all four of the parathyroids be removed before symptoms of underactivity develop?

Yes.

How soon after surgery upon the parathyroid glands can one do the following?

Get out of bed	Twenty-four to forty-eight hours.
Leave the hospital	Seven to nine days.
Bathe	Seven to nine days.
Return to normal activity	Four to six weeks.

48 *Peritonitis*

What is peritonitis?

Peritonitis is a bacterial infection of the peritoneal (abdominal) cavity.

What is the peritoneal cavity?

It is the free space within the abdomen surrounding the various organs, such as the stomach, intestines, gall bladder, appendix, liver, spleen, etc.

What are the most common causes for peritonitis?

a. Rupture of an abdominal organ, such as the appendix, small or large bowel, the gall bladder, etc.
b. Spread of infection from an inflamed organ, such as the Fallopian tube or ovary.
c. A wound of the abdominal wall which has extended into the peritoneal cavity, such as a gunshot or stab wound.

What are some of the symptoms and signs of peritonitis?

a. Pain in the abdomen.
b. Tenderness on pressure over the abdominal organs.
c. Loss of appetite, along with nausea and vomiting.
d. Distention of the intestines.
e. Temperature elevation.
f. Characteristic x-ray findings.

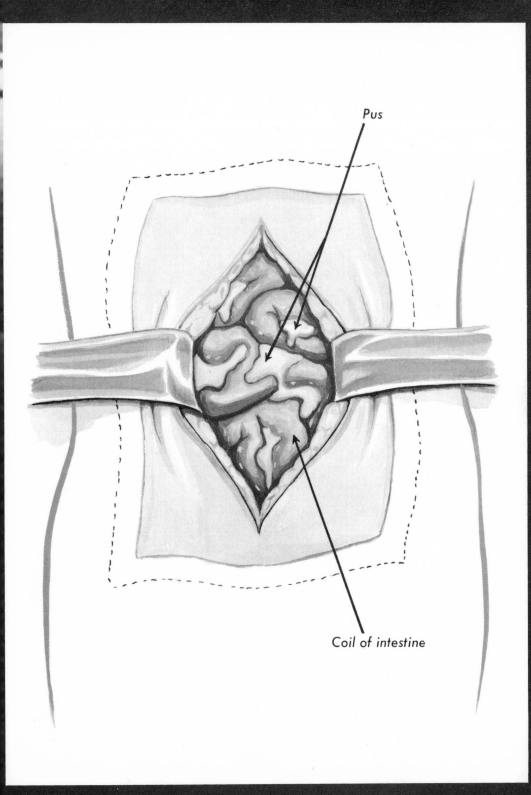

Pus

Coil of intestine

Peritonitis. This diagram shows peritonitis, a condition in which pus is present between the coils of intestine. Peritonitis is a most serious condition and requires surgery in order to eliminate the cause for the discharge of pus into the abdominal cavity.

Is peritonitis a serious condition?

Yes, as it results in severe toxemia. Untreated cases often lead to death because of overwhelming bacterial infection.

How can peritonitis be prevented?

a. By early attention to abdominal pain, with prompt treatment of the underlying condition. Appendicitis or acute gall bladder disease, if treated without delay, will not be complicated by rupture and consequent peritonitis.

b. Do not give laxatives to people with acute abdominal pain! Many an appendix has ruptured as the result of injudicious giving of a laxative.

c. Gonorrhea in the female should be treated early and strenuously. This will prevent the infection from spreading from the vagina into the uterus, Fallopian tubes, and out into the peritoneal cavity.

What are the methods of treating peritonitis?

a. Prompt surgery to remove the underlying cause, such as an acutely inflamed appendix or gall bladder.

b. Removal of pus from the peritoneal cavity by suction and the insertion of rubber drains which exit on the abdominal wall. This is to conduct to the exterior any new pus that may form.

c. If peritonitis is due to the rupture of an organ, such as the stomach, duodenum, or intestine, immediate surgery should be performed to repair the holes in these structures.

d. The giving of massive doses of the antibiotic drugs.

e. During the acute phases of peritonitis, a tube is inserted through the nose into the intestinal tract, to keep it free from distention, and the patient is fed intravenously.

What are the chances for recovery from peritonitis?

With the institution of prompt and adequate surgery, and the administration of large doses of antibiotics, the chances for recovery are excellent.

How long does it take for recovery from peritonitis to take place?

This will vary according to the cause of the peritonitis, the type of bacteria involved, the length of time it was in existence before active treatment was begun, and how far it has spread throughout the peritoneal cavity. Early cases of peritonitis may subside within a week, others of long standing may require several weeks for the patient to recover.

Are there any permanent after-effects of peritonitis?

Recovery is usually complete, but in some instances extensive adhesions may form. They may cause intestinal obstruction for weeks, months, or years after the acute process has subsided.

Physical Therapy
and Rehabilitation

49

What is physical therapy?

It is that branch of medicine which aims toward full restoration of strength and function to sick or injured structures, and toward aiding the convalescent to complete recovery. Physical therapy employs light, heat, electricity, water, and other mechanical agents in order to restore activity to an injured part of the body.

What is rehabilitation?

Rehabilitation employs physical agents in conjunction with attempts at psychological adjustment, social adjustment, and vocational retraining for handicapped people. Rehabilitation is directed not only toward the permanently handicapped but also toward the temporarily injured or ill patient.

LIGHT THERAPY

How is light used in the treatment of patients?

Ultraviolet light rays are used quite extensively in the treatment of certain skin diseases.

Should ultraviolet light rays be used without a doctor's supervision?

No. This is a dangerous procedure, as severe burns and damage to tissues may result from their improper use.

Do the ultraviolet lamps sold in drugstores deliver much ultraviolet ray?

These are usually inferior instruments and do not deliver the type and quantity of ray required for adequate therapy. However, they are not without dangers, as burns to the eyes, skin, and other structures can result from their overuse.

HEAT THERAPY

In general, how does heat help an injured part?

It has two main beneficial effects:
a. It increases the blood supply to the injured area, thus permitting nature to better heal the injury.
b. It relaxes spasm of blood vessels and muscles, thus promoting normal healing processes.

Are there different forms of heat therapy?

Yes. There are several types, with varying degrees of penetrative powers.

What are some of the instruments used for heat treatments?

a. An ordinary baking lamp. This does not have great penetrative powers but will help to a certain degree in improving circulation and in relaxing spasm.
b. Infrared machines. Infrared rays have some penetrative power but do not go deep into the tissues.
c. Diathermy machines, both long wave and short wave. These have considerable penetrative power and send heat waves into the substances of muscles, tendons, bones, etc.
d. Conductive heat. This is a type of heat in which there is direct conduction from the heat source into the body tissues. Hydrotherapy, hot baths, moist or wet dressings, and other procedures fall into this category.

Is it safe to employ heat treatments without medical supervision?

No. Whenever heat therapy is used, it should be prescribed by a

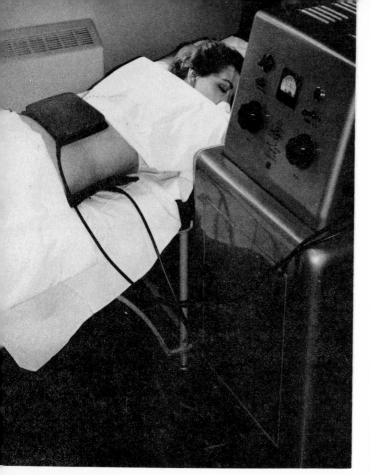

Left: Patient Receiving Diathermy Treatment. Diathermy sends dry heat beneath the skin into the muscles and deeper structures of the body. It is helpful in some cases of inflammation of muscles and joints. Home diathermy treatments are not without danger, as serious burns may result from misuse.

Below: Patient Receiving Hydrotherapy. Hydrotherapy in the form of whirlpool baths is helpful in improving the circulation to the limbs and in bringing heat to the muscles and joints. Hydrotherapy has also been beneficial in cases of paralytic poliomyelitis.

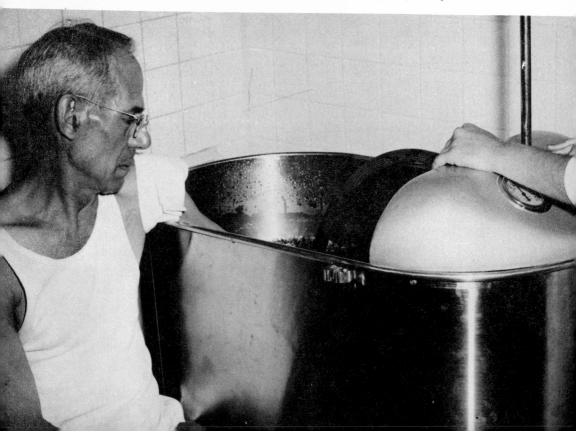

physician. Severe burns can result from the improper use of heat, whether it is merely in the form of a hot-water bottle or whether it is short-wave diathermy. Furthermore, the patient is not in a position to know when heat is the proper form of therapy or whether it will actually be harmful in certain conditions.

What types of illness or injury are aided by heat therapy?

These are so numerous that it would be impossible to enumerate all of them. A few of them are:

a. Arthritis of certain types.

b. Bursitis, during some of its stages.

c. Muscle sprains or inflammation.

d. Muscle spasm, as in poliomyelitis (the Sister Kenny treatment).

e. Stiff joints, tendons, and muscles, following prolonged immobilization, as after fractures.

How often do heat treatments have to be given to be effective?

They should be given almost daily over a period of several weeks to have their best effect.

ELECTRICAL STIMULATION

Is electricity used very often as a form of treatment in cases of neuritis or paralysis?

No. Electrical stimulation will not cause a damaged or paralyzed nerve to return to normal.

What are the most frequently used types of electrical stimulation?

Galvanic and faradic current. These can be applied by a specially devised machine.

How is electrical stimulation used as a form of treatment?

By stimulating a muscle to contract during the period that its nerve is not functioning properly, it is often possible to keep the muscle in better tone.

Will the giving of electrical treatments cause a facial paralysis to heal more quickly?

Probably not. This condition is a self-limited one and the rate of recovery of the nerve will not depend to a very great extent upon electrical stimulation.

Is the application of electrical stimulation helpful in making the diagnosis of disease?

Yes. It is extremely helpful in distinguishing the cause of the nerve paralysis or muscle degeneration.

HYDROTHERAPY

What is hydrotherapy?

It is a form of physical therapy utilizing water.

What are the benefits of hydrotherapy?

Swimming tanks, whirlpool baths, hot sprays and hot tub baths are all excellent for relaxing spasm and increasing the blood supply to various areas of the body.

Is hydrotherapy valuable as an after-treatment for poliomyelitis?

Yes. Swimming relaxes muscles and allows those which have poor function to be used more effectively. It is amazing to note the improvement in motion when a partially paralyzed patient is put into a tank of water and allowed to swim about.

Will whirlpool bath treatments aid a fractured part to return to normal function more quickly?

Yes. Such treatments tend to relax spasm and allow for more active motion in stiff muscles, joints, and tendons.

Are whirlpool baths beneficial in treating sprains, strains, lumbago, etc.?

Yes.

MASSAGE

Is it safe for a patient to have himself massaged without a doctor's prescription?

No. Much harm can come from improper massage, as muscles and joints can be damaged by too strenuous and too conscientious a masseur.

When is it bad to use massage?

a. When it is used to bring about weight reduction. Massage, by itself, does not lead to weight loss.

b. Where there is a lump or mass present. This may be a tumor, and massage can do it great harm.

c. Massage is contraindicated in an area of pain or inflammation. Massaging an area of inflammation may cause the infection to spread.

d. It is perhaps best not to massage emotionally unstable people. (Such persons tend to depend upon massage instead of facing reality and solving their problems through psychotherapy.)

What information should be given to the physiotherapist before massage is undertaken?

It should be stated whether the massage is to be deep or light, whether it is to be carried out in order to stimulate or in order to quiet down muscles, tendons, and joints.

What are the beneficial effects of properly administered massage?

a. It tends to relax muscles.

b. It tends to increase motion of joints, muscles, and tendons.

c. It tends to increase the blood supply to the area.

EXERCISE

Are exercises valuable in the treatment of bone, muscle, joint, and other diseases?

Most definitely, yes. Properly prescribed exercises can do a tremendous amount of good for conditions involving the muscles, bones, joints, tendons, and nerves.

Are there specific exercises which will aid specific conditions such as a slipped disc, lumbago, wry neck, and for illnesses such as cerebral palsy, muscular dystrophy, etc.?

Yes. Expert medical attention by specialists in this field will often result in great improvement in the above conditions.

Can anyone prescribe exercise, or should one go to a specialist in the field?

This has become a highly specialized field, and the various types of apparatus and exercises to be used should be prescribed by an expert in this field of medicine.

Is it necessary for exercises to be conducted frequently and under controlled conditions?

Yes. Most failures in physical exercises are the result of an improperly prescribed program or infrequent exercise periods.

REHABILITATION

What are the goals of rehabilitation?

a. To restore the patient to as near-normal a physical condition as possible.

b. To improve the patient's emotional state, so that he makes the best of his situation and adjusts to his handicap.

c. To improve the patient's social adjustment, so that he may resume his place in the community.

Have rehabilitation methods improved within the last fifteen to twenty years?

The advancement in this field has been one of the most remarkable in all of medicine. No longer do we think in terms of people being "crippled." Special institutions for rehabilitation have restored the

Right: Neck-Stretching Exercise for Neck Injury. For injuries such as a slipped disc, stretching the neck will often bring relief of pain. A single treatment will not bring permanent improvement; treatments should be given at regular intervals.

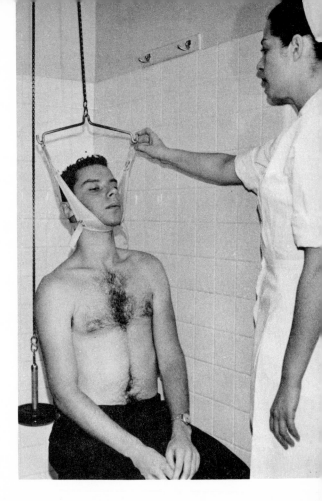

Below: Shoulder Wheel Exercise. Specialized exercises are valuable in aiding people to regain normal function of their muscles, tendons, and joints. This picture shows a patient using a revolving wheel to relieve stiffness in a shoulder joint.

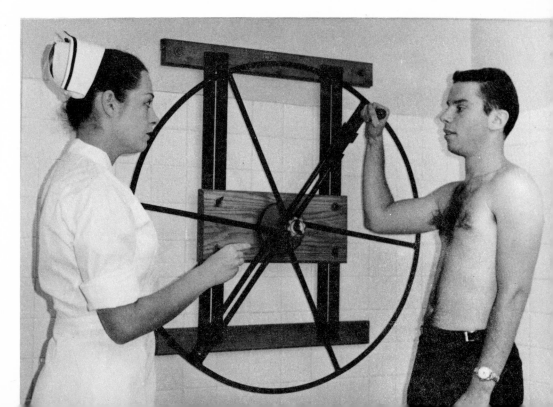

vast majority of handicapped people to a state wherein they are useful, productive, self-sustaining members of society.

For what types of illnesses are rehabilitation methods most valuable?

a. For the patient with a disabling birth deformity.

b. For the paralyzed patient.

c. For the patient with an amputation.

d. For the patient with incapacitating diseases of the nerves, muscles, bones, or joints.

e. For the patient who has partially recovered from a long and debilitating illness but who has not yet been able to resume normal physical, emotional, or social activity.

What percentage of those who have had prolonged illness will require some form of rehabilitation?

It is estimated that 5 per cent of all hospitalized medical patients and 80 per cent of all orthopedic patients need further care after their discharge from the hospital.

During what phase of illness is rehabilitation most needed?

During the convalescent period. It is extremely important that people who have recovered from serious illness should be encouraged to return to normal activity as quickly as possible. There is a tendency for many of the chronically ill to "adjust" to their illnesses and to display a lack of interest in returning to full activity.

Is there a tendency for people to accept their status as an invalid?

Yes. For some peculiar psychological reason, people who have been tended and cared for as total invalids for prolonged lengths of time have a tendency to accept their situation. Rehabilitation measures must therefore counteract this natural tendency and work upon people so that they desire to return to normal living, if this is possible.

What apparatus is used most frequently in order to bring about rehabilitation?

This cannot be answered by listing the names of various instruments or pieces of apparatus. A rehabilitation center will tailor apparatus so that it fits the particular need of the individual.

Can any physician or any hospital perform rehabilitation treatments satisfactorily?

No. Unfortunately, at this stage of our medical development, not all physicians and not all hospitals are equipped to do this work. It is much to the advantage of the patient to go to a rehabilitation center, where experts will use knowledge and instruments which are specific for the problem at hand.

50 *Pilonidal Cyst*

What is a pilonidal cyst?

It is an irregularly shaped cyst located in the lower back just above and between the cheeks of the buttocks.

What is the cause of these cysts?

It is thought that they are caused either by a defect in the development of the embryo or by ingrown hairs which become encysted.

How frequent are pilonidal cysts?

Almost 5 per cent of all people have pilonidal cysts.

Do these cysts tend to be inherited or to run in families?

No.

How is it that these cysts rarely evoke any symptoms until early adult life?

Hair grows within these cysts, and this may take a long time. Eventually, however, it is common for infection to take place within the cyst, and then pus will form and the patient will become aware of a pain in the region.

How can one know if he has a pilonidal cyst?

By the formation of a lump between the buttocks, by a yellowish

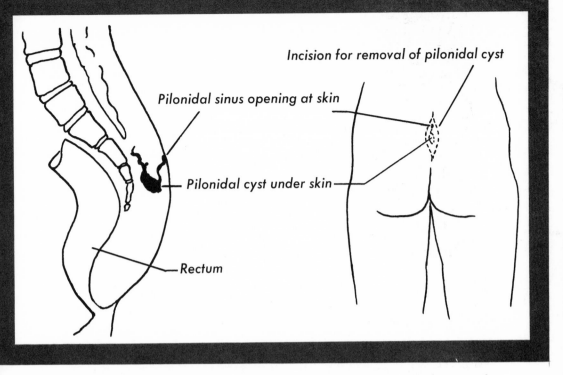

Pilonidal sinus opening at skin

Incision for removal of pilonidal cyst

Pilonidal cyst under skin

Rectum

Pilonidal Cyst and Incision for Its Removal. This diagram shows the location of a pilonidal cyst and outlines the incision made to remove the cyst. Pilonidal cysts are encountered frequently in young adults and are thought by most investigators to be birth deformities. Other, more recent investigators feel that they are caused by ingrown hairs.

discharge which appears from time to time on the underwear, and often by pain, tenderness, and abscess formation in the region.

How does the physician make the diagnosis of pilonidal cyst?

There are one or more small openings in the skin which lead into the cyst. From these openings, one often sees hair protrude and, when infected, pus will exude through these openings.

What are the harmful effects of a pilonidal cyst if not treated?

a. The cyst may become markedly enlarged and may tunnel in several directions for a distance of several inches.

b. There may be a chronic discharge and discomfort in the region.

c. An abscess may form which will cause extreme pain and high temperature.

d. In rare instances, these cysts may turn into malignant growths.

Is there any way to prevent the development of a pilonidal cyst?

No.

What is the treatment for pilonidal cyst?

Surgical removal.

How is the surgical treatment carried out?

By wide excision of the skin, subcutaneous tissue, and the entire cyst-bearing area extending down to the tissue overlying the sacral bone. Most surgeons pack these wounds wide open and permit them to fill in gradually from the bottom. A few surgeons close the skin tightly after removing the cyst, but this method is followed by recurrence in a large percentage of cases.

Are operations for pilonidal cysts serious?

No. They are considered to be minor operative procedures.

What type of anesthesia is used?

Spinal, or in rare instances, a local anesthetic such as novocaine is given.

Are there any special preoperative or postoperative measures which are necessary?

No.

Is there a great deal of postoperative discomfort?

Yes. A moderate amount of pain will be felt in the operative area. Also, there may be some discomfort because of inability to move the bowels for a few days after the removal of a pilonidal cyst.

Will bowel function eventually return to normal after this operation?

Yes, within a few days.

How soon after the removal of a pilonidal cyst can the patient get out of bed?

The day following surgery.

How long a hospital stay is usually necessary?

Approximately five days to one week.

Are these wounds often packed and left open?

Yes.

Does the packing have to be removed?

Yes. Usually within four to six days.

Is it painful when the packing is removed?

Yes.

What special postoperative routines are advised after the removal of a pilonidal cyst?

Tub baths, frequent changes of the dressings, visits to the surgeon's office every few days, and the maintenance of cleanliness in the area.

How long does it take these wounds to heal?

Anywhere from four weeks to four months, unless they have been closed tightly at surgery. The latter type of case may have complete healing within two weeks, but the chances of recurrence are much greater.

Does one have to remain out of work throughout the entire time the wound is healing?

No. Many patients can return to work within two to three weeks after this operation. However, they will have to make frequent visits to their surgeon's office for change of dressing.

Is there a tendency for these pilonidal cysts, once removed, to recur?

Yes, in approximately 2 to 5 per cent of all cases.

For how long must one be wary of recurrence after an apparently successful operation?

Recurrences have been noted as long as one to two years after surgery.

What is the treatment for recurrence?

Reoperation, making sure to leave the wound wide open so that it fills in solidly from the bottom.

How soon after a pilonidal operation can one do the following?

Bathe	Four to seven days.
Walk out in the street	Five to seven days.
Drive a car	Two to three weeks.
Return to work	Three weeks.
Resume marital relations	Three to four weeks.
Resume all normal activities	As soon as the wound has healed completely.

51

The
Pituitary Gland

What is the pituitary gland, and where is it located?

It is a small, nut-sized endocrine gland, measuring about one-half inch in diameter, located at the base of the skull underneath the brain. It is divided into two parts, the anterior and the posterior portion, each of which contains different types of cells and secretes different types of hormones into the bloodstream.

What hormones are secreted by the pituitary gland, and what are their functions?

a. The anterior portion of the pituitary secretes several hormones which influence the activity of the other endocrine glands such as the thyroid, the adrenals, the ovaries, the testicles, the breasts, and the pancreas. Secretions from the anterior pituitary regulate and control the activity of these above-mentioned glands, sometimes stimulating them to greater activity, at other times inhibiting their activity. For instance, if the adrenal gland is low in secreting its hormone into the bloodstream, the anterior pituitary hormone will stimulate it toward greater secretion.

b. The posterior pituitary manufactures a hormone which controls the retention and excretion of water from the kidneys.

Do endocrine glands such as the adrenals, thyroid, etc., ever influence the activity of the anterior pituitary?

Yes; as an example, when the adrenal secretion reaches the desired

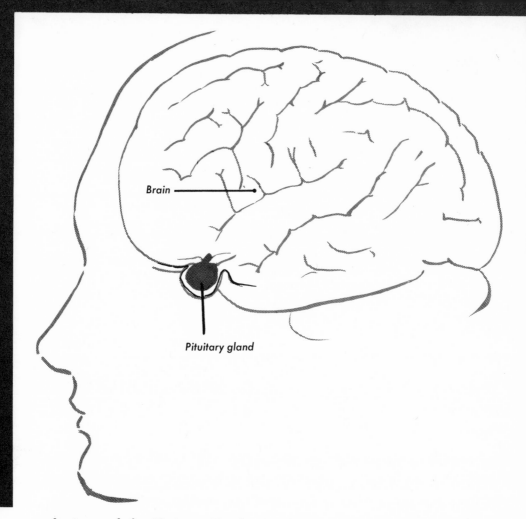

Brain

Pituitary gland

Anatomy of the Pituitary Gland. This diagram shows the pituitary gland as it nestles within the bony structure of the skull. A tumor within the pituitary gland will press upon the optic nerves which supply the eyes and this may lead to impairment of vision.

level, it will act to inhibit the pituitary from producing more of its secretion.

What other hormone does the anterior pituitary gland secrete?

It secretes a hormone responsible for growth and development.

Is the pituitary gland referred to as the "master gland"?

Yes, because it appears to control the function of all the other glands within the body.

1008

Does the pituitary gland often undergo tumor formation?

Yes. Pituitary tumors account for approximately 10 per cent of all growths within the skull and brain.

What takes place when the anterior portion of the gland becomes overactive and undergoes tumor formation?

Two conditions may result:
a. If certain cells within the anterior pituitary become too active, overstimulation of the adrenal glands will result and Cushing's disease develops.
b. If other cells within the anterior pituitary become overactive, an excess of growth hormone will be produced and giantism or acromegaly will result.

How can a definite diagnosis of a pituitary tumor be made?

In addition to the clinical symptoms which develop, there are characteristic changes noted on x-rays of the skull. The pituitary gland is nestled in a bony cavity called the sella turcica, and when the gland has undergone tumorous growth the edges of this bony cavity become eroded.

What are the characteristics of giantism?

When the anterior pituitary produces excessive quantities of its growth hormone during childhood before bone development is complete, the individual grows to an enormous size. This condition is responsible for the giants we see who are seven or eight feet tall.

Is there a tendency for giantism to be inherited?

No. Whereas there is a very definite tendency for size to be inherited, the abnormal conditions resulting in giantism are not inherited.

What are the characteristics of acromegaly?

If there is an overproduction of the growth hormone in adult life, after bone structure has been fully developed, then height and the length of the extremities are not altered. However, there is tremendous overgrowth of certain bony parts of the body, such as the hands, the feet, and the features of the face. This results in a characteristic distortion of the facial features.

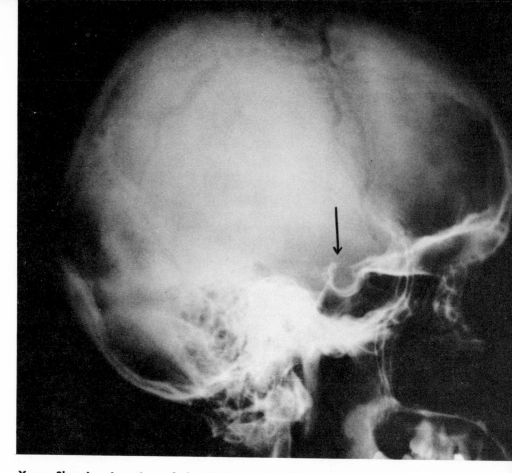

X-ray Showing Location of the Pituitary Gland. Destruction of the small bones which surround the pituitary gland can be seen on x-ray when a tumor is growing within the gland. Most pituitary tumors can be controlled successfully either by x-ray therapy or by surgical removal of the gland.

What other changes take place as a result of excessive growth hormone secretion?

The body chemistry is altered and severe muscular weakness, cessation of menstrual periods, impotence, and even diabetes may ensue.

What is the treatment for giantism or acromegaly?

The disease process often stops by itself. If it progresses, x-ray radiation of the pituitary gland is carried out, and if this is ineffective, surgical excision of the gland is performed.

How successful are x-ray therapy and surgery in halting excess pituitary activity?

In most instances, these forms of treatment will arrest the process.

Can a normal child who appears to be small in stature be made to grow taller by the giving of pituitary hormones?

No. At the present time, there is no effective method of stimulating greater growth in normal children by the giving of pituitary extracts.

Is there any effective way to stimulate growth in a child who appears to be undersized?

If the small size is due to undernourishment, to lack of good hygienic conditions, or to underactivity of some of the other glands such as the thyroid, growth may be stimulated by correcting such deficiencies.

Is there any safe and effective way of stopping a child from growing too tall?

No.

Are there any disease states which result from underactivity of the pituitary gland (hypopituitarism)?

Yes. If underactivity occurs in childhood, growth will be retarded markedly. Children so affected will remain small but well proportioned. They retain a childlike appearance throughout life. This condition is responsible for the little dwarfs one sees at a circus.

If underactivity of the pituitary commences during adulthood, growth cannot be stunted. However, such a situation will lead to a depression in the function of all the other endocrine glands, such as the thyroid, the adrenals, the ovaries, and the testicles.

Is pituitary dwarfism inherited?

No. If pituitary dwarfs marry and have children, they usually have normal-sized children.

What are some of the other symptoms of hypopituitarism?

Weakness, general apathy, loss of energy, and, in some cases, mental disturbance. The skin takes on a wrinkled appearance as seen in old age. There may be lowering of the blood sugar and loss of appetite and weight.

What is the treatment for underactivity of the anterior pituitary?

If the condition is due to a tumor of the pituitary, then x-ray therapy or surgery may be helpful. Medical treatment will consist of replacement of the deficient hormones by injection or oral medication.

Can the serious effects of underactivity of the anterior pituitary be counteracted by treatment?

Yes, to a certain extent, but cure is not often possible.

What is the function of the posterior portion of the pituitary gland?

The production of a hormone which acts upon the kidneys so as to prevent them from excreting too much water.

What is diabetes insipidus?

It is a condition caused by too little production of hormone by the posterior pituitary and adjacent nerve tissue. It leads to a serious chain of events in which the kidneys can no longer control the amount of water they excrete.

What are some of the characteristic symptoms of diabetes insipidus?

Since the kidneys excrete huge quantities of water, the patient must drink incessantly in order to maintain sufficient amounts within his body.

Can diabetes insipidus be treated effectively?

Yes. There are available potent extracts of the posterior pituitary gland which can be given to the patient by injection or as a snuff. However, the condition is not curable and the patient must continue to receive these injections for the rest of his life.

Is there any relationship between diabetes insipidus and so-called "sugar diabetes"?

No.

Are diseases of the pituitary gland preventable?

No.

SURGERY OF THE PITUITARY GLAND

What are the indications for operating upon the pituitary gland?

When it has been determined that it has undergone tumor formation. This may be evidenced by the onset of progressive loss of vision, headache, changes on x-ray showing erosion of the bone around the gland, or by the onset of signs such as are seen in Cushing's disease and acromegaly or giantism.

Is surgery upon the pituitary gland safe?

An operation involving the pituitary gland is a serious one; nevertheless, it is reasonably safe.

Where is the incision made to approach the pituitary gland?

Except in bald people, the incision is made almost completely within the hairline. In any event, the scar resulting from surgery is inconspicuous.

What are the chances for recovery from an operation upon the pituitary?

About 90 per cent.

Is the pituitary gland usually removed completely when it is the site of tumor, or is it sufficient to remove it partially?

In most cases, an amount sufficient to relieve pressure on the nerves concerned with vision is removed.

How successful are operations for pituitary tumors in relieving symptoms?

As a rule, operations for pituitary tumors are undertaken because of tumor formation with progressive loss of vision. Therefore, the visual status before operation is an important consideration. Generally speaking, most patients are considerably improved following operation, provided too much damage had not occurred preoperatively.

How is a decision made as to whether to treat a pituitary tumor with x-ray or with surgery?

Although opinions vary on this point, x-ray treatment is usually tried first unless vision is already seriously impaired. If vision continues to fail despite x-ray treatment, surgery is indicated.

If there has been impairment of vision due to a pituitary tumor, will surgery upon the gland restore vision?

In most cases, yes.

How long a hospital stay is necessary following operations upon the pituitary gland?

Usually about ten days to two weeks.

How long do these operative procedures take to perform?

About two to three hours.

Do tumors of the pituitary gland ever recur once they have been removed?

Yes, in a small percentage of cases. Such people may then be treated by x-ray therapy or they may be reoperated.

Do tumors of the pituitary gland often spread to other parts of the body?

No. This happens extremely rarely.

Can one lead a normal mental life after a pituitary operation?

Yes. One's mental state is not affected by tumors of the pituitary gland.

Are operations upon the pituitary followed by paralysis of any of the limbs?

No.

Can acromegaly be cured by pituitary surgery?

No, but the process can be halted from progressing further.

Will the bony overgrowths and appearance return to normal after surgery in acromegaly?

Unfortunately, no.

52 *Plastic Surgery*

*(For specific surgery, see the chapter
on the organ involved.)*

What is plastic surgery?

A branch of surgery devoted to the restoration, repair, and correction
of malformations of tissues. It is concerned not only with return to
normal *appearance*, but also with restoration to normal *function*.

What is the difference between cosmetic surgery and plastic surgery?

Cosmetic surgery aims toward improving or restoring the *appearance*
of tissues or organs, such as the nose or the breasts. Plastic surgery,
while including cosmetic surgery, goes much further than this, as it
aims toward restoring and improving *function* as well as appearance.

**What parts of the body and what conditions are most commonly oper-
ated upon by plastic surgeons?**

It is commonly thought that plastic surgery is limited to operations
upon the face. This is not the actual case. A partial list of conditions
for which plastic surgery is performed includes:

   a. Surgery of the nose (rhinoplasty).

   b. For lop ears.

   c. To remove ugly scars anywhere on the body.

   d. For receding chin.

   e. For harelip.

f. For cleft palate.

g. For restoration of eyelids or external ear.

h. Plastic operations upon the breasts.

i. For excessive fat on the abdomen (lipectomy).

j. For skin contractures.

k. For burns anywhere on the body.

l. Skin grafting anywhere on the body.

m. For removal of skin blemishes, skin cancers, skin tumors.

n. For deformities of the male or female genitals.

Is it necessary to go to a plastic surgeon in order to have plastic surgery performed?

Yes, for most conditions requiring specialized knowledge.

Is special training necessary for a physician to become a plastic surgeon?

Yes. Most plastic surgeons are first trained as general surgeons and then receive additional years of education, learning the special art of plastic surgery.

What is the difference between plastic surgery and restorative surgery?

Restorative surgery is a branch of plastic surgery which attempts to return injured parts to normal function.

Are the results of plastic surgery usually permanent?

Yes, unless an operation has been performed in an attempt to slow down aging processes, such as an operation to remove skin wrinkles. In such cases, as the patient ages, there is a tendency for a recurrence.

Should plastic surgery be performed upon children, or is it wiser to wait until they have attained maturity?

Plastic surgery is quite successful when performed on children. However, it is better to wait for a growing part, such as a nose, to attain its full development before correcting its appearance.

In performing plastic surgery, what tissues of the body may be used as grafts?

    a. Skin lends itself excellently toward being used as a graft.

    b. Cartilage from ribs is often used as a graft to build up a sagging nose.

    c. Bone transplants are also used as grafts, as in operations to fuse the spine or to build up the hip joint.

    d. The cornea has been used successfully as a graft to restore lost eyesight in certain selected cases.

Can a plastic surgeon always predict the outcome of an operation he is going to perform?

With reasonable certainty, although he cannot always predict the *exact* appearance that will result. Much will depend upon the peculiar healing characteristics of the individual patient.

Can a plastic surgeon tell in advance how skin will heal and whether the scars will be smooth or ugly?

Not always. Certain people have a tendency to heal with almost invisible scars; others heal with thick, overgrown scars.

SKIN GRAFTS

What are skin grafts?

They are portions of skin used to cover areas which have been laid bare by burns, by injuries, or by surgical removal of diseased tissues.

Does skin taken from one person work satisfactorily when grafted to another person?

No. These grafts are almost always unsuccessful, except when they take place between identical twins.

Are grafts usually successful when portions of skin are taken from one part of the body and grafted to another part of the body?

Yes, if performed under the proper circumstances.

1017

If a part of the body, such as a finger or an ear, has been completely severed from the body, can it be grafted back on to the body?

These procedures are usually unsuccessful, although in the rare case such an operation has proved successful if it was performed immediately after the injury and if the severed part had been kept relatively clean.

What are the various types of skin grafts?

a. Pinch grafts. These are small pieces of skin, averaging about one-quarter inch in diameter, made up of the superficial layers of the skin. A dozen or more of these grafts may be taken from a donor area and placed at spaced intervals as small islands in the recipient site. They often grow well in their new location and spread out so as to fully cover the bare area.

b. Split-thickness grafts. These are sheets of the superficial and part of the deep layers of the skin which are removed from the donor area by a special knife. This type of graft is usually taken from a flat surface of the body, such as the abdomen, the thigh, or the back. They are most useful as a covering for large burned areas where the skin has been completely lost, as in a third-degree burn. These grafts will take if the recipient site is free of infection and appears to be healthy.

c. Full-thickness grafts. These contain all the layers of the skin but not the underlying subcutaneous tissues. They are of the greatest value when they are used on weight-bearing recipient areas which are subject to a great deal of wear and tear. Full-thickness grafts are cut so that they exactly match the recipient area.

d. Pedicle grafts. These are grafts in which one portion of the skin remains attached to the donor area while the rest is transplanted to the recipient area. A pedicle graft will retain its own blood supply, which comes into it from its attached portion. The pedicle, or base of the graft, is detached from its original site when the free part of the graft develops its own new circulation at the recipient site. These grafts are most useful in covering defects about the face where a wide area of skin has been removed. A pedicle graft may also be used to cover an entire finger or hand.

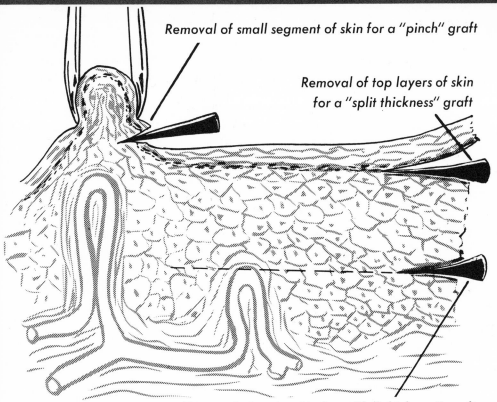

Removal of small segment of skin for a "pinch" graft

Removal of top layers of skin for a "split thickness" graft

Removal of entire skin for a "full thickness" graft

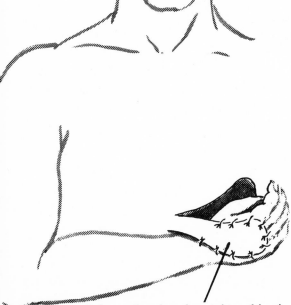

Pedicle graft taken from skin of body and grafted on to back of hand

Skin Grafts. This diagram shows a "pinch graft," wherein just a small segment of skin is lifted out from one part of the body and placed over a raw area elsewhere; a "split-thickness graft," which takes a segment of the upper layers of the skin; a "full-thickness graft," which removes all the layers of the skin; and a "pedicle graft," in which a segment of skin is partially detached from one area and attached to another part of the body.

1019

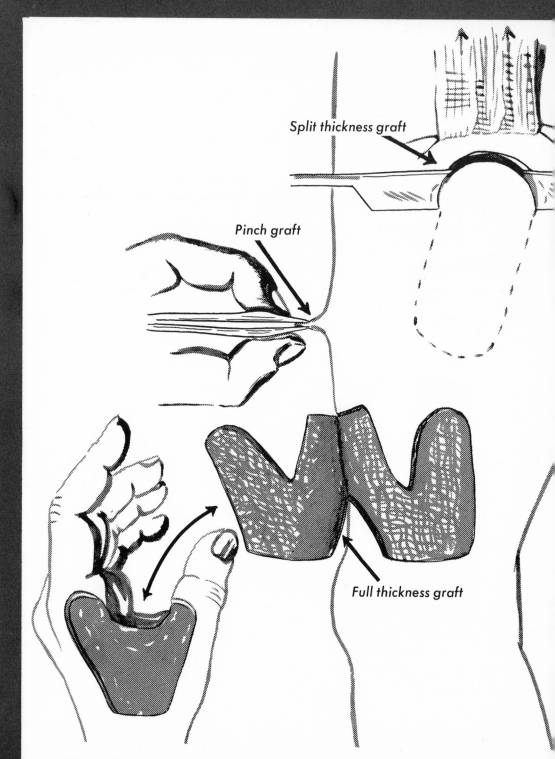

Split thickness graft

Pinch graft

Full thickness graft

Skin Grafts. Grafts will not grow unless the sites to which they are to be attached are healthy and free of infection. Grafts from one person to another are rarely successful.

What determines whether a graft will be successful?

a. The donor site must be clean and free of infection.

b. The recipient site must be clean and free of infection.

c. The recipient site must have good blood supply.

d. The graft must be applied evenly and smoothly.

e. The graft must always be in firm contact with the recipient site.

f. Measures must be taken to see that the graft does not become detached from the recipient site once it has been placed there.

g. Grafts must be applied without tension or undue stretching.

h. The general health of the patient must be good, so that healing will take place normally.

How soon can one tell whether a skin graft has taken?

Usually, the dressings at the recipient site are changed a week to ten days after the graft has been applied. It will not be known until that time whether the graft has been successful.

Will grafted skin have sensation in it?

For several weeks there may be a numb feeling in the region; eventually, normal sensation will come to a grafted area.

Will hair grow in grafted skin?

Not unless it is a full-thickness graft which grew hair in its original site.

Is it possible to transplant skin containing hair from one part of the body to another and have a growth of hair at the recipient site?

Although some hair may grow, it will not resemble the hair at the recipient site. (This cannot be done successfully on the scalp.)

Is grafted skin sometimes of a different color than the skin which had originally been there?

Yes. Also, grafted skin does not necessarily assume the color of the new area. For this reason, surgeons will attempt to graft skin of the same shade when it involves a visible area such as the face or the neck.

1021

Is grafted skin as strong and resistant as normal skin?

The pinch grafts and the split-thickness grafts are usually not as strong as normal skin. Full-thickness grafts, however, will eventually be almost as strong as normal skin.

Is it important to prevent grafted skin from getting a severe sunburn?

Yes. Grafted skin seems to be somewhat more sensitive to the rays of the sun.

If grafts are unsuccessful, is it possible to perform the operation over again?

Yes. Split-thickness grafts can be taken from the same donor site when it has healed completely.

For what type of skin lesions is plastic surgery frequently advocated?

a. Ugly, disfiguring scars.

b. Keloids (overgrowth of scar tissue).

c. Contractures of the skin, usually secondary to old burns.

d. Bare areas secondary either to third-degree burns or to the surgical removal of large portions of skin.

Can thick, unsightly scars be converted into thin, fine linear scars?

Yes. By excising the old scar, undermining the subcutaneous tissues, and repairing the skin edges with plastic techniques, ugly scars can often be almost completely eliminated.

What determines the need for a skin graft when performing the removal of a skin lesion?

If the edges of the wound cannot be brought together readily or if too much tension is created by attempting to suture the skin edges, the surgeon may decide to fill in the bare area with a graft.

Pregnancy and Childbirth

THE PRENATAL PERIOD

Are classes of instruction for prospective parents available?

In nearly every community in the country, classes are made available for both prospective mothers and fathers. In these classes, the anatomy, physiology, and complications of pregnancy are discussed. Such classes are extremely useful and will help to relieve fears which some young people have about the experience of becoming parents. It is just as important for the prospective father to attend these classes as for the mother.

What are the symptoms of pregnancy?

a. The most consistent symptom is a missed menstrual period.

b. Enlargement of the breasts and tenderness of the nipples, occurring within the first few weeks of pregnancy.

c. Increased frequency of urination within the first few weeks of pregnancy.

d. Nausea and vomiting, known as "morning sickness." This symptom may begin during the second month of pregnancy. Actually, the symptoms are not limited to the morning, but may occur at any time.

e. In later pregnancy, abdominal enlargement becomes apparent.

f. Movements of the baby, known as "feeling life," start between the fourth and fifth month of pregnancy.

1023

Do these symptoms always indicate pregnancy?

No. Some of these symptoms may be found with other conditions. However, when these symptoms are correlated with specific physical findings, the diagnosis of pregnancy is easily made.

How soon after the onset of pregnancy can the obstetrician make a positive diagnosis?

At approximately the time of the *second* missed menstrual period, that is, after four to six weeks of pregnancy.

What are the characteristic physical signs of pregnancy?
a. Enlargement and softening of the uterus.
b. Bluish discoloration and softening of the cervix.
c. Brownish discoloration of the area around the nipples.
d. After the fourth or fifth month, the baby's heartbeat may be heard by listening with a stethoscope placed on the mother's abdomen.
e. An x-ray of the abdomen will show the skeleton of the fetus after the fourth or fifth month.

Is a missed menstrual period always indicative of pregnancy?

No! A hormone imbalance, a debilitating disease, or severe emotional upset may occasionally cause a woman to miss a menstrual period.

Does menstruation occur during pregnancy?

No. Menstruation is a term applied to regular bleeding from a non-pregnant uterus.

Is vaginal bleeding always considered to be abnormal when the uterus is pregnant?

Yes. Even very early bleeding is abnormal and, in most instances, is associated with a threatened miscarriage.

In very early pregnancy, can a menstrual period be brought on by medication?

No! Even in early pregnancy, medications will not induce bleeding.

In cases where the missed period is due to causes other than pregnancy, bleeding may be brought on by any one of several medications.

Is it necessary to take a careful medical history of a pregnant woman?

Yes. This is very important, and such a history should include a complete family and personal history. Such familial conditions as diabetes, tuberculosis, twins, etc., are important to know as soon as a woman becomes pregnant. Also, the history of previous surgery or previous serious medical illness, such as a cardiac condition, a kidney condition, or allergic disease, is extremely important to note.

Why is it so important to take a careful medical history?

Because the presence of one of the above conditions may influence the obstetrician to alter his management of the pregnancy and its subsequent delivery.

What are some other important medical conditions which should be known about a pregnant woman?

a. Previous pelvic infection.
b. A history of infertility.
c. The woman's correct age, as well as her husband's age.
d. Previous obstetrical history.

What kind of physical examination should be conducted upon a pregnant woman?

A complete physical examination, including thorough investigation of the heart, lungs, breasts, abdomen, and pelvis. The patient's blood pressure and weight should be checked at each prenatal visit. The importance of these findings will become apparent when toxemias of pregnancy are discussed.

What laboratory tests should be performed?

a. A complete blood count.
b. A complete urine analysis.
c. An examination of the blood for syphilis.
d. An examination of the blood to determine the Rh type.
e. A chest x-ray.

Is an x-ray of the pelvis necessary?

Not as a routine procedure. Where there is some question, after examination, about the size and shape of the bony pelvis or the size of the baby's head in relation to the pelvis, an x-ray examination is indicated.

If x-rays are indicated, when is it best to take them?

Just before, or at the onset of, labor.

Must all pregnant women be examined internally?

Yes! There is no substitute for a thorough internal examination. Abnormalities of the uterus, tubes, ovaries, or bony pelvis can be detected most readily by a pelvic examination.

Is there a danger of miscarriage following an internal examination?

Certainly not!

Why do some obstetricians perform a pregnancy test rather than an internal examination?

In cases where the patient is extremely apprehensive or has had previous miscarriages, an obstetrician may be forced to delay his internal examination and to rely upon a laboratory test simply because the "patient's ignorance" might erroneously blame the internal examination for any subsequent, but unrelated, vaginal bleeding.

Can the obstetrician tell during an early examination if a Cesarean section will be necessary?

Not usually. First examinations are usually performed to determine the presence of pregnancy and to rule out pelvic abnormality. Examinations at this time may or may not be extended to determine the size and shape of the bony passageway. Many obstetricians delay this part of the examination until the seventh month. Except in markedly deformed and obviously inadequate pelves, the necessity for Cesarean section does not become apparent until the end of pregnancy or the onset of labor.

How does the obstetrician determine when the baby is to be born?

The most common method is to count 280 days from the beginning of the last regular menstrual period.

How accurate can the obstetrician be in determining the date of the baby's birth?

The obstetrician's prediction will usually be accurate within a two-week range from the date of the child's birth.

Should the patient make the choice of the hospital in which to be delivered?

No. The patient should use the hospital in which her obstetrician has full privileges. A wise patient will permit her obstetrician to select the hospital.

Is there any such thing as a normal pregnancy diet?

Yes. The diet should be a balanced one with approximately fifteen hundred to two thousand calories. The diet should be high in proteins, minerals, and vitamins, with a moderate amount of carbohydrates and a minimum of fats, salt, and spices.

What specific items are important to include in pregnancy diets?

Milk, eggs, cheese, meat, poultry, green vegetables, garden vegetables, and fruits.

How much weight should the average pregnant woman gain?

No more than fifteen to twenty pounds for the entire pregnancy.

Should vitamins be taken during pregnancy?

In a well-balanced, controlled diet, extra vitamin intake is not necessary. However, because of the eating habits of most people today, it is perhaps best to take supplementary vitamins in order to counteract any possible deficiency.

Should iron be taken during pregnancy?

Yes, when some degree of anemia exists. Some investigators believe that the routine use of iron throughout pregnancy will prevent the onset of anemia.

Is anemia a common occurrence during normal pregnancy?

Yes.

Why must salt intake be limited during pregnancy?

The intake of salt in large quantities results in the retention of fluids in the tissue spaces. It has been found that such retention of fluids is closely related to the toxemias of pregnancy. (See the section on Complications of Pregnancy in this chapter.)

Is it safe for a pregnant woman to drink alcoholic beverages?

An occasional cocktail, highball, or glass of beer is not harmful. Excessive intake of alcohol is harmful both to the baby and to the mother.

Is smoking permitted during pregnancy?

Yes, but in moderation. Heavy smoking during pregnancy is harmful both to the baby and to the mother.

What restrictions on physical activity should be imposed upon pregnant women?

The normal pregnant woman may engage in all of the usual physical activities as long as she is able to do so without discomfort. As pregnancy progresses, her ability may decrease. Very strenuous or excessive physical activity should be curtailed at all times.

Is bending, stretching, or raising the arms harmful during pregnancy?

Absolutely not! This is an old wives' tale and has no truth whatsoever.

What is the best clothing to wear during pregnancy?

a. A good brassière is essential to support the enlarging breasts.

b. A firm girdle will give the patient a feeling of support and relieve some of the lower abdominal or lower back or thigh discomfort which sometimes accompanies the later months of pregnancy.

c. Low or medium heels should be worn. This is particularly important, as there is a tendency to slip and fall during the later months of pregnancy—and high heels are conducive to such accidents.

d. A garter belt should be used to support stockings. *Elastic garters around the legs or thighs should never be worn!*

Why are elastic garters not to be worn?

Because they may produce varicose veins.

Is bathing permitted during normal pregnancy?

In the early months of pregnancy, tub baths or showers are permitted. In the later months, showers are preferable over tub baths, as stepping into and out of a tub may lead to falls.

Is ocean bathing or pool bathing permitted during pregnancy?

Yes, until the seventh month. Care should be taken to stay away from rough water and to avoid too strenuous activity, such as diving.

What special care should be given to the breasts during pregnancy?

a. A good supporting brassière is essential.

b. If the nipples are retracted, an attempt to bring them out should be made. This is done by grasping the nipple gently and pulling with a slight rotating movement in an outward direction.

c. Where there is a discharge from the nipples, cotton or gauze pads should be used as a protective measure.

d. Nipples should be washed regularly with a mild soap.

Are pregnant women permitted to travel in an automobile, train, or plane?

Yes, except when there is the threat of miscarriage, as evidenced by vaginal bleeding or abdominal cramps.

Is miscarriage ever caused by a bumpy automobile, train, or plane trip?

No. This is a common misconception with no scientific substantiation.

Should pregnant women drive automobiles?

Yes, until the eighth month. After that time, because of their increased girth and a tendency toward delayed physical reaction, it is advisable not to drive.

Is sexual intercourse permitted during pregnancy?

Yes, until the end of the seventh month. However, if there has been any vaginal bleeding, intercourse should be avoided.

Why is intercourse not permitted during the last two months of pregnancy?

Because of the possibility of introducing infection into the vaginal canal.

How often should a pregnant woman visit her obstetrician?

Throughout the first six months, a visit every four weeks is indicated. During the seventh and eighth months the patient should visit the doctor every two or three weeks, and then once a week for the last four weeks. Women should not hesitate to phone or visit their obstetrician at any time, should a complication arise!

Why are regular, periodic visits important during pregnancy?

To spot the onset of complications at the earliest possible time, and to prevent them in some instances. Weighing the patient, taking her blood pressure, examining the urine, listening to the baby's heartbeat, judging the growth and development of the baby, etc., are helpful ways of making sure that everything is going well. Also, a regular visit will offer an opportunity to answer the mother's questions, to reassure her, and to allay any unfounded fears.

At what stage of pregnancy does the abdomen become visibly enlarged?

Usually, after the third month. At the fifth month, the top of the uterus is at the level of the navel. At the eighth month, the top of the uterus reaches the bottom of the breastbone. In the ninth month, the baby settles in the pelvis and the abdomen looks slightly smaller again.

Should the pregnant woman take extra rest periods?

Yes, as most pregnant women are easily fatigued.

Is douching permitted during pregnancy?

No, because of the danger of introducing infection into the uterine cavity.

How soon after the onset of pregnancy does the mother "feel life"?

Fetal movements, or "quickening," are first noticed about the fifth month after the last menstrual period. At first, these are just faint, fluttering movements, but later, actual marked movements can easily be felt by placing a hand upon the abdomen.

Can the baby's movements be felt every day?

Not necessarily. Nor are they felt all day long. In many instances, only occasional movements are felt once or twice during the course of a day.

What is "lightening"?

It is a term applied to the sensation which occurs when the baby's head drops into the pelvis. In first babies, this occurs about three weeks before labor begins. After the first baby, this may not occur until labor actually starts.

Can a mother tell when "lightening" takes place?

Yes, sometimes. There is a feeling of more breathing space and the mother notes a lowering of the height of the abdomen. She may also feel increased pressure within the pelvis and greater difficulty when walking.

When does the obstetrician usually take pelvic measurements?

Pelvic measurement is performed either at the first visit, or, more commonly, about six weeks before the expected date of confinement. This is done by vaginal and rectal examination.

What information does the obstetrician obtain from such an examination?

a. The general size of the various planes of the pelvis, such as the inlet, the mid-pelvis, and the outlet.

b. The configuration or bony type of pelvis.

c. Any abnormalities in the soft tissues or bones in the region.

Are instruments used in this pelvic measurement?

Not necessarily. The obstetrician, by experience, using his fingers and hands alone, can frequently make an accurate determination of the size of the pelvis. Old-fashioned methods of measuring external points, such as the crest of the pelvic bone and the base of the pelvic bone, have been abandoned as having little or no relation to the actual size of the inside of the bony pelvis.

Can the obstetrician determine, beforehand, if labor will be easy or difficult?

No. The obstetrician can tell only if the pelvis is adequate or inadequate. He can also tell whether the baby is in the right position or if there is a pelvic abnormality.

The kind of labor the mother will have is an unknown factor. A good strong labor can overcome most difficulties. Even a large baby can come through the average pelvis without harming the mother or damaging itself.

Must the obstetrician always take x-rays of the pelvis?

No. This is done only when he feels that there is some question about the adequacy of the pelvis or when there is concern about the position or size of the baby.

What is the treatment for the nausea and vomiting of pregnancy (morning sickness)?

a. In the presence of repeated attacks of nausea and vomiting, all restrictions on diet are lifted and the patient is permitted to eat anything she desires.

b. Innumerable preparations, including antispasmodics, antacids, vitamins, sedatives, etc., have been given to treat this condition. Newer drugs include the antihistaminics and the tranquilizers.

c. Severe cases which fail to respond to ordinary measures may have to be hospitalized and treated with intravenous feedings to restore fluid and mineral balance. Most of these women have an underlying psychological problem and may require treatment by a psychiatrist to tide them over this difficult period.

Is the cause for "morning sickness" known?

No.

Are all cases of nausea and vomiting due to emotional disturbances?

No! However, these factors will make it difficult for the patient to accept the average discomfort which accompanies early pregnancy.

Is it common for pregnant women to have excess production of saliva?

Yes. This is a frequent complaint, often replacing nausea and vomiting. Small doses of atropine will relieve this condition. Also, the chewing of hard candy or chewing gum will help the patient to swallow the saliva.

Is special care of the teeth necessary during pregnancy?

Yes. Proper oral hygiene must be exercised. A sufficient amount of calcium must be included in the diet. This is usually obtained by the drinking of milk and the eating of cheese. For people with poor teeth, extra calcium and vitamin C are given in tablet form.

Should women receive active dental treatment during pregnancy?

Yes. Dental care can be carried out throughout all of pregnancy without the fear of precipitating a miscarriage. However, it is best not to take a general anesthetic without the consent of the obstetrician.

How is constipation treated during pregnancy?

By eating those foods which tend toward regularity. Fresh and stewed fruits, bran cereals, and buttermilk should be included in the diet. If these measures are unsuccessful, mild laxatives may be used. Mineral oil is to be avoided, since it may interfere with digestive processes.

Are hemorrhoids a frequent complication of normal pregnancy?

Yes, particularly in the later months. They are caused by the pressure of the baby upon the large veins in the pelvis.

What is the treatment for hemorrhoids during pregnancy?

a. Rectal suppositories to relieve pain.

b. Medications to soften the stool.

c. The application of witch hazel or ice packs to the anal region if pain is severe.

d. The application of anesthetic ointments in the presence of severe pain.

e. When a large hemorrhoid has clotted and produces severe pain, it may be necessary for a small incision to be made in order to evacuate the blood clot.

Should hemorrhoids be removed during pregnancy?

No.

What causes frequency of urination during pregnancy?

a. Pressure of the enlarging fetus upon the dome of the bladder.

b. Infection of the bladder (cystitis).

What is the treatment for frequency of urination?

a. If frequency is due to pressure of the baby, the mother can do very little about it.

b. When the frequency is due to infection, active treatment is carried out by giving of sulfa drugs or antibiotics.

Are varicose veins of the legs very common during pregnancy?

Yes. These are due to back pressure upon the pelvic veins by the enlarging uterus.

What is the treatment for varicose veins during pregnancy?

a. Any constricting garters must be immediately removed.

b. An elastic bandage encircling the entire leg or elastic stockings should be used to give even support to the veins of the extremity.

Is surgery advocated for varicose veins during pregnancy?

No.

Do varicose veins ever disappear after delivery?

Many of them will disappear or become much smaller. Each subsequent pregnancy may cause an aggravation, both in the symptoms and in the size of the varicosities.

Is it natural for women to have a vaginal discharge during pregnancy?

Yes. Some slight increase in vaginal secretion is entirely normal. However, an erosion of the cervix or a fungus infection of the vagina may cause discharge associated with an itch in the region of the vulva. Such conditions should be treated during pregnancy.

Are douches used to treat vaginal infections during pregnancy?

No. They are not used, because of the danger of extending the infection into the uterine cavity.

What causes backaches during pregnancy?

The most common cause is the change in posture which is adopted to compensate for the enlarging abdomen. In other words, the patient attempts to change her center of gravity.

What is the treatment for backache?

The use of a firm girdle or support will tend to relieve most backaches. However, some discomfort may be noted despite all measures.

What causes leg cramps during pregnancy?

a. A change in posture which places a new kind of tension upon leg muscles.
b. The failure of the body to absorb sufficient calcium.

How are leg cramps treated?

a. Immediate relief can often be obtained by standing on tiptoe and bending the knees, or by pressing the toes against the end of the bed or against a wall.

b. If cramps are due to insufficient calcium, calcium and antacid tablets will frequently control them.

What causes the heartburn so frequently noted during pregnancy?

It is usually caused by excess stomach acidity and is seen most commonly in the later months of pregnancy. It is associated with belching and a sour taste in the later months of pregnancy. Persistent heartburn or indigestion should be reported to the obstetrician, as in a small proportion of cases these symptoms may be early signs of toxemia.

What is the treatment for heartburn in pregnancy?

The simplest remedy is to take small sips of milk. If this is unsuccessful, antacid powders or similar preparations should be taken. (Antacids containing bicarbonate of soda should be avoided.)

What causes swelling of the feet, ankles, or other parts of the body during pregnancy?

a. Pressure on pelvic veins. This is usually noticeable after standing for several hours and is relieved by rest in bed. Such swelling has no clinical significance.

b. Varicose veins. Such swelling is treated by the use of elastic bandages or stockings.

c. Toxemia of pregnancy. In such conditions, the swelling is not restricted to the lower extremities but may appear in the fingers, the face, the back, or the abdominal wall. When associated with the finding of albumin in the urine or elevated blood pressure, drastic steps must be taken to relieve the condition.

What is the cause of dizzy spells during pregnancy?

In early pregnancy, particularly in hot or humid weather, dizziness or fainting spells are rather common and are not considered serious. In the later months of pregnancy, if they are associated with other symptoms, such as tissue swelling, spots before the eyes, or nausea and vomiting, they may be an evidence of toxemia of pregnancy.

LABOR

(Delivery and Confinement)

What is the usual normal mechanism of delivery?

The most normal mechanism is one in which the baby's head comes first. This is called vertex (head) presentation, and the head is termed the leading or presenting part.

Can the obstetrician determine what part of the baby is going to come first?

Yes, by examining the abdomen.

What parts other than the head sometimes present themselves just before or at the onset of labor?

The buttocks or legs may come first. This is called breech presentation. Occasionally, a baby's arm or shoulder will be the presenting part. Such a situation will complicate delivery. Sometimes, the baby's head, instead of being bent toward its chest, is extended or bent backward. This then becomes a face or brow presentation. This, too, constitutes a complication of delivery.

What causes abnormal presentation?

In many instances, the cause is unknown. In other cases, it is caused by:

a. Abnormal shape of the mother's pelvis.

b. Tumors, such as a fibroid of the uterus.

c. Placenta praevia, in which the afterbirth is implanted beneath the level of the baby's head.

d. Abnormalities of the baby itself.

What is done when the baby is found to be in an abnormal position?

The treatment for abnormal position depends upon many factors, such as:

a. The number of pregnancies the woman has already had.

b. The type of abnormality encountered.

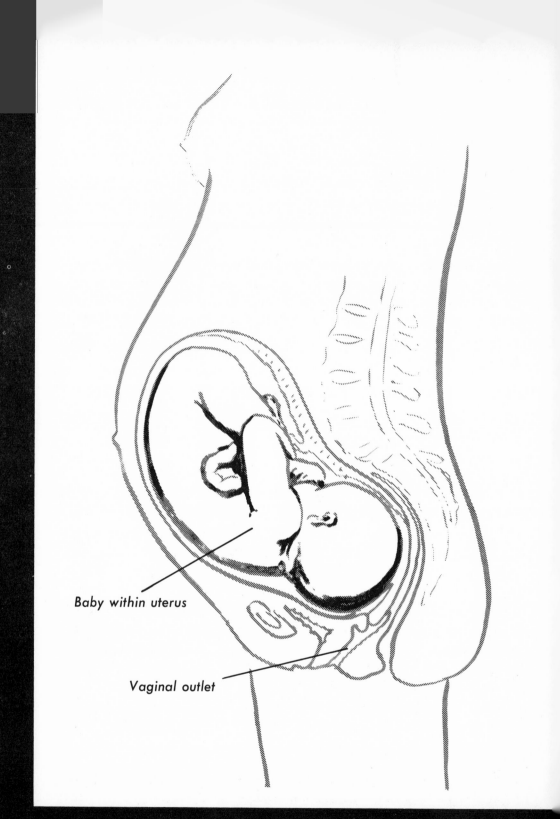

Baby within uterus

Vaginal outlet

Head Presentation during Labor. This is the most common of all positions. During labor, the head molds so that it conforms to the contour of the inner aspect of the

   c. The presence or absence of active labor at the time of discovery of the abnormal position.

   d. The stage of labor present when the abnormal position is encountered.

   e. The presence or absence of ruptured membranes.

   f. The size of the baby.

   g. The general condition of the mother.

All of these factors will influence the obstetrician in deciding what course to take. Some abnormal positions spontaneously convert to normal as labor progresses; others can be assisted by the obstetrician to return to normal presentation. Some babies may be delivered without complication, even with the abnormal presentation. Finally, in certain instances, the obstetrician may resort to Cesarean section to carry out delivery.

How can a woman tell when labor is beginning?

Labor begins any one of three ways:

   a. Abdominal pains or contractions.

   b. Rupture of the bag of waters.

   c. Staining from the vagina.

How are these signs identified?

Contractions or pains are identified by a feeling of tightness in the abdomen, with discomfort in the back radiating around to the front, or pain high in the abdomen radiating down toward the pelvis. There may also be a tight feeling in the thighs. In early labor, contractions are irregular and last for only a few seconds. After a few hours, the contractions come closer together, last longer, and are more painful. When the bag of waters breaks, there may be just a little trickle of fluid or a big gush may ensue. If the bag of waters breaks before contractions have begun, the contractions will usually follow within twenty-four hours. When staining occurs, contractions usually follow within twenty-four to forty-eight hours.

What are the various stages of labor?

   a. The first stage is calculated from the onset until complete dilatation (opening) of the cervix or mouth of the womb.

1039

b. The second stage begins at the time of complete dilatation of the cervix and ends with delivery of the baby.

c. The third stage begins with the delivery of the baby and ends with the delivery of the placenta, or afterbirth.

How long does normal labor last?

In first babies, the average duration of the first stage of labor is approximately eighteen hours. After the first baby, the average duration of the first stage is less than eight hours.

In first babies, the second stage of labor lasts about one hour. After the first baby, the second stage is usually less than an hour.

The third stage of labor usually lasts only a few minutes but occasionally continues as long as one hour. The modern obstetrical trend is to cut the third stage of labor as short as possible by removing the afterbirth quickly.

What is meant by "false labor pains"?

In the later months of pregnancy, the muscles of the uterus are extremely irritable and may undergo frequent contractions. These contractions resemble labor only in that there is a sense of tightening. False labor pains have no effect on dilating the cervix or pushing the baby downward.

Is it ever necessary to treat false labor pains?

Yes. Sedatives are sometimes given to lessen the awareness of these annoying contractions.

When should the patient starting labor go to the hospital?

This is a variable factor and depends upon each obstetrician's method of management. Some of the important considerations are:

a. The further the patient lives from the hospital, the sooner she should depart for it.

b. If it is the first baby, it will probably be longer in coming and the patient can take more time before departing for the hospital.

c. Patients with known abnormalities or complications of pregnancy should be hospitalized earlier than others.

At what stage of labor is hospitalization mandatory?

With the first baby, when good strong contractions occur every five minutes for one full hour. With subsequent pregnancies, depending on the distance from the hospital, when contractions are occurring every ten to fifteen minutes.

Is it always better to go to the hospital early?

Not necessarily. In normal pregnancy, it is better for the patient to stay at home until labor is well established. If there have been previous pregnancies and there is a history of rapid labor, it is perhaps better to leave for the hospital earlier than usual.

INDUCED LABOR

What is meant by "labor by appointment" or "induced labor"?

This is a method of initiating labor artificially at, or near, full term. It is done in some cases because of a medical condition such as high blood pressure, toxemia, etc. In other instances, it is practiced in women who have had previous pregnancies. When properly carried out in suitable cases, it can be accomplished without harm to baby or mother.

What are the advantages of induced labor?

a. The mother comes to the hospital in the morning, after a good night's sleep. She can fast before coming to the hospital, so that her stomach is empty prior to delivery.

b. She can make arrangements before she leaves for the hospital to have her other children taken care of.

c. Her husband can arrange his affairs so that he is at the hospital during labor.

d. The doctor can schedule the labor at a time when he is free of office hours or other duties which might keep him from attendance.

e. The hospital staff is alert and fully staffed during the daytime hours when labor is being induced.

f. All hospital activities, such as those that take place in the blood transfusion department, the x-ray department, the laboratories, the operating rooms, the delivery rooms, etc., are fully staffed and ready to carry out any necessary procedure during the day hours.

Can all patients be delivered by induced labor?

No! Certain conditions must be present before artificial induction of labor is advised. These are:

a. The patient must be at, or near, the regular time for delivery (not sooner than thirty-eight weeks after the onset of pregnancy).

b. The baby should be in a normal position of presentation, with the head down in the pelvis.

c. The cervix should be soft, thinned out, and slightly open.

If the above conditions are met, there are no dangers to either mother or baby from induction of labor.

How is labor induced?

a. By artificially breaking the water bag with a sterile instrument. This is a painless procedure and requires no anesthetic.

b. By the use of pituitary extract injections to stimulate contractions of the uterus.

NATURAL CHILDBIRTH

What is natural childbirth?

This term refers to the method of management in which special care is taken to prepare the patient psychologically for pregnancy, including the prenatal period, labor, and the postpartum period (the period following delivery).

What are the aims of natural childbirth?

To banish unwarranted fears, thus preventing tension and in this way reducing pain to a minimum. The vicious cycle of fear-tension-pain is difficult to break once it has been established. If natural childbirth can do away with the element of fear, the vicious cycle is abolished.

How does natural childbirth work?

It is accomplished by a course of instruction in the mechanism of pregnancy and by establishing a closer relationship between the patient and the obstetrician. Also, the patient develops a familiarity with the hospital area and personnel so that the eventual labor and delivery will not take place in a strange atmosphere.

Why doesn't every patient have natural childbirth?

a. Not all patients are emotionally suited to natural childbirth.
b. Most obstetricians do practice some of the aspects of natural childbirth by trying to allay fear, by instilling confidence, and by encouraging the patient to read or attend courses given by various agencies for prospective mothers and fathers.

Must one take a formal course in natural childbirth?

Not necessarily, but most large communities do have such courses. They include visits to the hospital, lectures by hospital physicians and nurses, instructions in breathing exercises, and, in some instances, specific instructions as to what should be done when labor approaches.

Should the husband participate in natural childbirth?

Yes, so that he can be an emotional aid to his wife during times of expectant stress. In most institutions where natural childbirth is practiced, husbands are allowed to remain in the labor room with their wives during the first stage of labor.

Does natural childbirth mean delivery without sedatives or anesthesia?

Not at all! The patient is always aware of the fact that sedatives are available if she or her obstetrician thinks they are necessary. Anesthesia is also available if needed. However, the patient who practices natural childbirth and is emotionally prepared for labor will require a minimum of both sedatives and anesthesia. The patient should feel no shame or disgrace if she needs assistance from these agents. Natural childbirth is not an endurance contest!

What are the advantages of natural childbirth?

a. A better understanding of the role to be played in pregnancy.
b. A more relaxed, emotionally stable attitude throughout pregnancy.
c. Less discomfort, as a result of understanding and relaxation.
d. A sense of well-being and active participation in the most natural of all human phenomena.

Are there any advantages to the baby in natural childbirth?

Yes. The baby is often more alert at birth, breathing and crying takes place spontaneously and is not delayed, and there is more chance for a spontaneous delivery because of the ability of the mother to assist during the second stage of labor.

Why is the baby more alert during natural childbirth?

Since the mother has received less in the way of sedatives and anesthesia, the unborn child is not affected by these medications. It must be remembered that any medication given to the mother will affect the child as long as the child is within the mother's body.

What are the disadvantages of natural childbirth?

The only disadvantage arises in the patient who is emotionally unsuited for the experience. Such patients may build up more tension than normal by hiding their fears, and thus they will defeat the primary aim of natural childbirth.

❉   ❉   ❉   ❉

What happens when the patient reaches the hospital in labor?

In most institutions, after registering at the desk, the patient is accompanied by an aide to the labor floor. She is then admitted to a labor room, undressed, and given a gown or short jacket to wear. If she is in active labor, she is examined immediately by her own obstetrician, if he is present, or by one of the hospital residents or internes. This examination determines the stage of labor that she is in.

The pubic region is then shaved and, if the situation permits, an enema is given.

Is the obstetrician always notified immediately upon admission of a patient to the hospital?

Yes. The obstetrician is always contacted by the interne or resident as soon as the exact stage of labor has been determined.

What other tests are performed upon the patient, following hospitalization?

The blood pressure is taken, a sample of urine is examined, and the baby's heartbeat is listened to and recorded. A blood count is taken and the patient is given a physical examination of the heart and lungs by the house physician. A history is either taken by the house physician or supplied to the hospital records by the obstetrician—from his office charts.

How is the progress of labor determined?

By frequent rectal examinations. This will show the extent of dilation of the cervix and the position of the presenting part of the baby.

Who performs examinations upon the patient during labor?

Examinations are performed by the obstetrician, the house physician, and in some smaller institutions by obstetrical nurses who are experts in the field.

Is frequent examination during labor important?

Yes. This is the only way to note the progress of labor and to spot any abnormality, should it develop.

Should the obstetrician be in attendance throughout all of labor?

With first babies, this is not necessary, and in most recognized hospitals throughout the country the obstetrician is expected to visit his patient only periodically. During the first stage of labor, the patient is observed by the house physicians and nursing staff. If labor is rapid and progressing quickly, the obstetrician will naturally

1045

remain within easy reach of the labor floor. With second or subsequent babies, because of the shorter labor, most obstetricians remain on the labor floor or in the hospital throughout the entire course of labor.

When is medication given for relief of pain?

In the earlier stages, before labor is well established, most obstetricians will administer a mild sedative, such as a barbiturate. This will allow the patient to relax and permit labor to progress unhampered. When labor is well established and contractions are frequent, stronger drugs, such as demerol, may have to be given to relieve intense pain. These drugs are to be used sparingly but may be repeated from time to time if labor is prolonged. Other drugs, such as the tranquilizers or antihistamines, have been used effectively to supplement the use of pain-relieving drugs and to afford relaxation and relief from tension.

Is there any danger in the use of these drugs?

Not when they are used properly and under careful supervision.

Is the baby affected by narcotics or other drugs given?

Yes, but the effects have usually worn off by the time delivery occurs. This is the reason the proper timing of drug administration is so important. Where large doses of sedatives and narcotics have been given, the baby is sleepy and under the influence of these medications at delivery, and may require active resuscitation.

What are the effects of large doses of these medications upon the mother?

If the mother is too heavily under their influence, she may be unable to assist in the important second stage of labor, when bearing down and helping are so important.

What is "twilight sleep"?

It is a state of sedation or narcosis in which the patient can respond to instructions, assist when told to do so, and may experience some discomfort, yet has no memory of the condition after labor is completed.

How is "twilight sleep" brought about?

By the combination of drugs such as demerol and scopolamine.

What types of anesthesia are used in delivery?

a. Local injection with novocaine of the skin of the perineum. This will allow the obstetrician to enlarge the opening with a surgical incision (episiotomy).

b. Pudendal block, the use of novocaine injected into a group of nerves in the perineum. This anesthetizes the area of the vagina so that an episiotomy can be performed painlessly.

c. Caudal epidural block, saddle block, or spinal anesthesia. These methods utilize novocaine or similar drugs which are injected into openings in the vertebral column in order to produce anesthesia in the region of the vagina and outlet.

d. Inhalation anesthesia. This will include such gases as nitrous oxide, cyclopropane, or ether, in conjunction with oxygen.

What determines the type of anesthesia which will be used?

Each type of anesthesia has its advantages and disadvantages, and every institution has anesthetists with special preferences. There are innumerable considerations in determining which anesthesia shall be used for an individual patient. Where there are expert anesthetists available, the decision should be left to them. The obstetrician will always confer with the anesthetist and state his preference for his patient.

The condition of the unborn child is as important a factor in determining anesthesia as the condition of the mother. For instance, premature babies do not tolerate inhalation anesthesias very well. In such a case, the mother may be delivered by a local block anesthesia or may be permitted to have a spontaneous delivery without any anesthesia at all.

How is the condition of the baby checked during labor?

a. By listening, at frequent intervals, to the baby's heartbeat. Irregularities in the baby's heartbeat is an indication that something is wrong.

b. The appearance of meconium (the contents of the child's bowel)

1047

in the vagina is an indication of fetal distress. This finding is correlated with the heartbeat, and together they form a picture of fetal difficulty.

What is the treatment for fetal distress?

This depends upon the stage of labor and the nearness to delivery. These factors are weighed by the obstetrician in deciding the proper immediate management of the delivery.

When is the baby born?

When the cervix is fully opened and the baby's head is stretching the vaginal opening, delivery is imminent.

What does the obstetrician do when the head is stretching the vaginal opening?

He enlarges the opening by making an incision along the edge of the vagina. This is called an episiotomy. The head, shoulders, and the rest of the body will then emerge. Such an eventuality is called a spontaneous delivery. Occasionally, pressure applied by an assistant who presses gently on the top of the uterus will hasten the delivery. If the baby does not exit from the vagina after this stage is reached, forceps are commonly employed. (See the section on Forceps Delivery in this chapter.)

What is the advantage of an episiotomy?

It prevents tearing of the vagina or perineum near or through the rectum.

When is an episiotomy performed?

Just before expected delivery, after the patient has been anesthetized.

When is the incision of an episiotomy repaired?

Immediately after delivery of the baby, while the patient is still under anesthesia.

How long does it take an episiotomy incision to heal?

It heals in a matter of a few weeks.

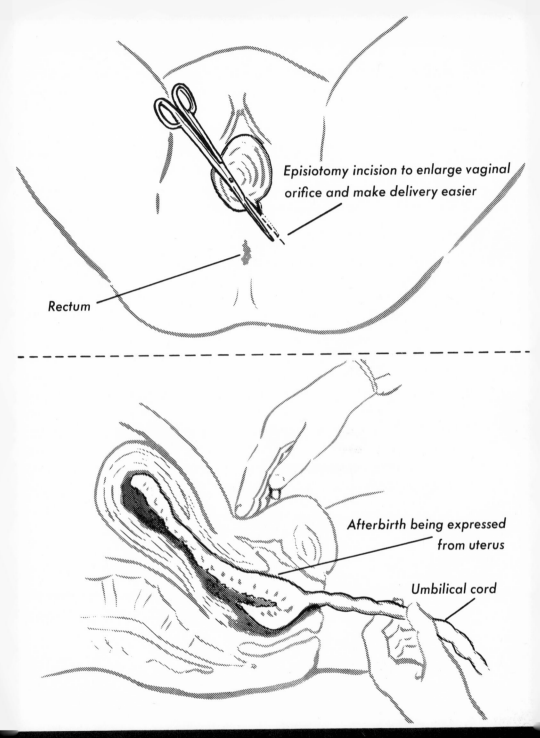

Episiotomy incision to enlarge vaginal orifice and make delivery easier

Rectum

Afterbirth being expressed from uterus

Umbilical cord

Episiotomy and Delivery of the Afterbirth. In order to prevent tearing as the head comes through the opening of the vagina, it is common practice for the obstetrician to make a surgical incision (episiotomy) in the vagina to allow more room for the child to emerge. This incision is repaired immediately after delivery.

The afterbirth is delivered by gentle pressure by the obstetrician over the uterus. This

Do stitches have to be removed from an episiotomy wound?

Usually not, unless silk stitches have been used.

Is an episiotomy always necessary?

In normal-sized babies with normal mothers, first labors almost always should be accompanied by an episiotomy. If the baby is a small premature one or the vaginal opening is unusually large, an episiotomy may not be necessary.

Is an episiotomy necessary after the first baby?

Where a previous episiotomy has been performed or where there is a rather sizable baby, episiotomy should be performed.

How is the afterbirth removed?

By gentle pressure on the uterus and gentle pulling on the cord. If any difficulty arises, it should be removed manually by the obstetrician, who inserts his hand into the uterus, separates the afterbirth carefully from the lining of the uterus, and removes it.

How is the baby separated from the umbilical cord?

At birth, the baby is placed on the mother's abdomen or on an adjoining table. The umbilical cord is then tied about one inch from the baby's abdomen and is cut across with a scissors.

FORCEPS DELIVERY

What are forceps?

In obstetrics, forceps are instruments used to help deliver the baby's head.

When are forceps used?

a. When the second stage of labor has been prolonged and the mother has been unable to push the baby out.
b. When the mother is tired and can no longer assist in the labor.
c. When the baby's head is not in the proper position to be delivered and must be rotated by the forceps.

d. When, because of one factor or another, the baby's head has not come completely through the pelvis to reach the opening of the vagina.

e. When signs of fetal distress appear and it is urgent to deliver the baby quickly rather than wait for natural processes to take their course.

Are forceps dangerous to the baby?

When used properly by a qualified obstetrician at the proper time and for a correct indication, forceps are not at all dangerous and cause no injury to the baby.

Delivery of a Baby's Head Assisted by Forceps. This is a photograph of an actual birth taking place with the aid of forceps. The forceps hasten and aid the smooth passage of the baby's head through the vaginal opening.

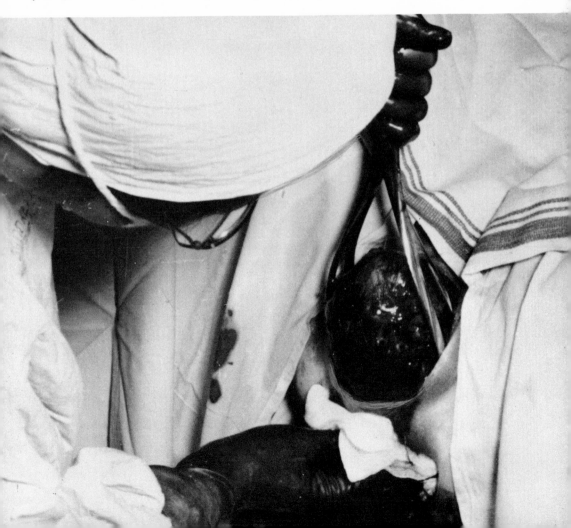

Are forceps dangerous to the mother?

No, unless used improperly.

Are there different types of forceps?

Yes. There are many types used for different purposes. Some are used to rotate the baby's head, some are used for traction on the head, others are used to exert traction in various directions to effect delivery of the head. Still others are used to deliver the head when the baby is in a breech position.

BREECH DELIVERY

What is a breech delivery?

One in which the baby's buttocks are delivered first.

Is breech delivery an abnormal situation?

In a certain sense this is an abnormal situation, but in the hands of a competent obstetrician, breech delivery can be carried out with safety to both mother and child.

How often does breech delivery take place?

In approximately 3 to 5 per cent of all full-term deliveries.

What causes breech presentation?

a. An abnormal pelvis.
b. Birth deformities of the uterus.
c. Fibroid tumors of the uterus.
d. Abnormality in the baby's head or tumor of the baby's head.
e. A placenta which is placed abnormally low within the vagina.
f. Twins.
g. An excessively large amount of fluid surrounding the baby.

If the first baby is a breech, will all other pregnancies be breech?

Not necessarily.

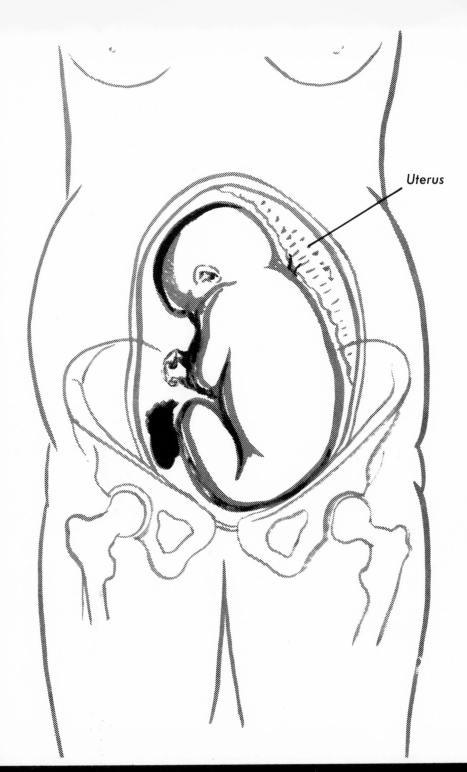

Uterus

Breech Presentation. This is less common than the head position, but most breech babies are delivered without too much difficulty. An infant presenting in this position will have less time for the head to mold to conform to the pelvic bones. Therefore children in breech position with large heads are sometimes delivered by Cesarean

At what stage during pregnancy does the baby assume a breech position?

This may not take place until actual labor has been established. It is not at all uncommon for the baby to change its position from day to day or even from hour to hour until the very terminal stages of pregnancy. Most breeches, however, are found at about the seventh month of pregnancy.

How is the breech position diagnosed?

a. By examination of the abdomen and noting that the head is in the upper part of the uterus.
b. By x-ray examination.
c. By vaginal examination during labor.

Can the breech position be corrected?

Some obstetricians advocate external rotation if the breech position is discovered before the onset of labor. However, other obstetricians believe that this should not be done as it may cause some harm. Furthermore, the baby may revert to the breech position even after it has been turned around.

How is breech position treated?

This is usually decided after the onset of labor. In first babies, the size and shape of the mother's pelvis must be accurately gauged, since the large diameter of the baby's head will not be shaped or molded during a breech labor. Therefore, such determinations must be made accurately before labor has progressed too far. If labor is good and the pelvis is adequate in size and the baby is not unduly large, labor is allowed to progress naturally. If labor is poor or the pelvis is inadequate in size or the baby is suspected of being large, a Cesarean section is indicated.

If a breech is found, should the patient go into the hospital at an earlier stage of her labor?

Yes, as the determination as to management must be made at an earlier stage of labor.

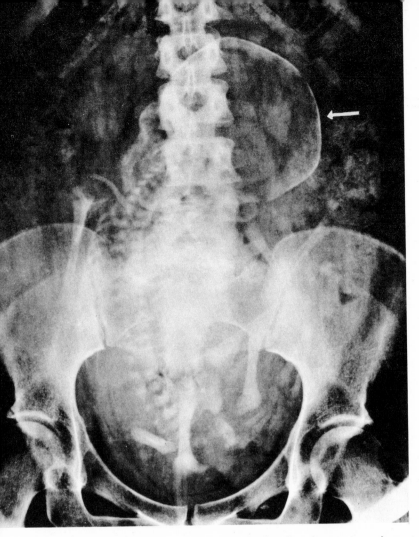

Baby's head

X-ray of Breech Position. Note that the head in this instance does not appear to be too large for the pelvis. This child delivered without difficulty through the vaginal route.

PROLAPSED CORD

What is a prolapsed cord?

It is a condition in which the umbilical cord drops down below the presenting part (the head or the breech) and comes through the cervix into the vagina. It may be only a partial prolapse, with the cord lying alongside the head, or a complete one in which the cord escapes through the cervix into the vagina all by itself.

How often does prolapsed cord occur?

In about one out of two hundred cases.

When is prolapsed cord seen most often?

After the membranes have ruptured in cases in which the baby is in an abnormal position.

Is there danger to the baby from a prolapsed cord?

Yes, since the circulation through the cord will be interfered with by compression between the bony parts of the baby and the mother. Such an interruption of circulation may cause the baby to die.

How is the diagnosis of prolapsed cord made?

a. By signs of fetal distress, such as slowing or irregularity of the heartbeat or presence of meconium in the vagina.

b. By the presence of the cord in the vagina or protruding from the vagina.

What is the treatment for prolapsed cord?

This will depend on the stage of labor and the closeness to delivery. In a mother having her third or fourth baby with good labor and a cervix almost fully open, a prolapsed cord can be treated expectantly since delivery will be imminent. Such a woman can usually be delivered from below. The patient is positioned with the legs and pelvis higher than the head, thus allowing the fetal presenting part to ease the pressure upon the cord. Oxygen is administered until time for delivery.

If delivery does not appear to be imminent, Cesarean section is carried out, providing there are still signs that the baby is alive and in good condition.

What emergency measures should be carried out if the cord prolapses while the patient is still at home?

The patient should be placed in bed, with her pelvis and legs elevated higher than the rest of her body. This can be accomplished by raising the foot of the bed on books. The doctor should be called immediately.

Is there any way to anticipate or prevent prolapse of the cord?

No.

MULTIPLE BIRTHS
(*Twins, Triplets, and Quadruplets*)

How often do twins occur?

About once in eighty cases.

How often do triplets occur?

About once in eight thousand cases.

How often do quadruplets occur?

About once in every seven hundred thousand cases.

What is meant by identical twins?

These are twins who have developed from one egg. These twins usually look exactly alike.

What are dissimilar twins?

They are those which have developed from two separate eggs. These twins may be of different sexes, and do not look any more alike than two brothers or two sisters or a sister and brother.

What causes twin births?

a. Identical twins result from the complete splitting of one egg after it has been fertilized.
b. Dissimilar twins result from the release of two eggs from the ovaries and the fertilization of each egg by a separate sperm.

Is the tendency toward multiple births inherited?

Yes.

Can multiple births occur when there is no family background of such births?

Yes.

When can twins or multiple births be diagnosed?

Usually after the fifth month of pregnancy.

How is the diagnosis of multiple births made?

By feeling more than one head on abdominal examination or by hearing more than one fetal heartbeat. Confirmation can be obtained by taking x-rays.

How does the obstetrical management of multiple births differ from that of single births?

The obstetrician will observe the patient more closely for signs of toxemia and for earlier labor because of the larger size of the uterus. A patient with twins or multiple birth is usually admitted to the hospital at an earlier stage in labor.

How is labor of multiple births managed?

The presentation of the first baby is determined and the patient is managed accordingly. Most babies will deliver head-first. The second most common situation is one in which one baby delivers head-first and the other by breech presentation. X-rays are used to determine the position of each baby.

INERTIA LABOR

What is inertia labor?

It is a condition characterized by poor contractions of the uterus. Inertia labor may be primary, that is, the contractions may be poor from the very start; or it may be secondary, that is, after a prolonged period of good labor, the pains become weak and ineffective.

What are the causes of inertia labor?

Primary inertia may develop in an overdistended uterus, such as one containing a very large baby or twins, or it may develop in those uteri which have too much fluid. Tension and fear may also play a role in the causation of primary inertia.

Secondary inertia is caused by prolonged labor, dehydration, and exhaustion of the mother. This situation arises when the mother's pelvis is not adequate for the size of the baby's head or when some abnormal presentation exists. In other cases, it is caused by failure of the cervix to dilate.

What is the treatment for inertia labor?

Assuming that the presentation is normal, the pelvis is adequate, and the baby's head has entered the mother's pelvis, inertia is treated primarily with medications to stimulate the uterus to contract regularly and more forcefully. Pituitary extract is given to increase uterine contractions, the patient is given sufficient quantities of fluids to combat dehydration, and sedatives are administered to release tension. If some abnormality is present, such as abnormal position of the baby, this may involve performing a Cesarean section.

CESAREAN SECTION

What is a Cesarean section?

It is an operation devised to deliver a baby surgically by an incision in the abdomen and then into the fundus of the uterus.

Is Cesarean section a major operation?

Yes.

How often are Cesarean sections performed?

In about 4 per cent of all deliveries in the United States.

Is Cesarean section a safe procedure?

Yes. In normal women, the recovery rate is close to 100 per cent. Where some complication of pregnancy exists, the recovery rate is somewhat lower. With the present knowledge and skill developed in surgical technique and anesthesia, along with administration of blood and the use of antibiotics, Cesarean section has become an extremely safe surgical procedure.

When was Cesarean section first performed?

It is thought that it was performed first in the fifteenth century

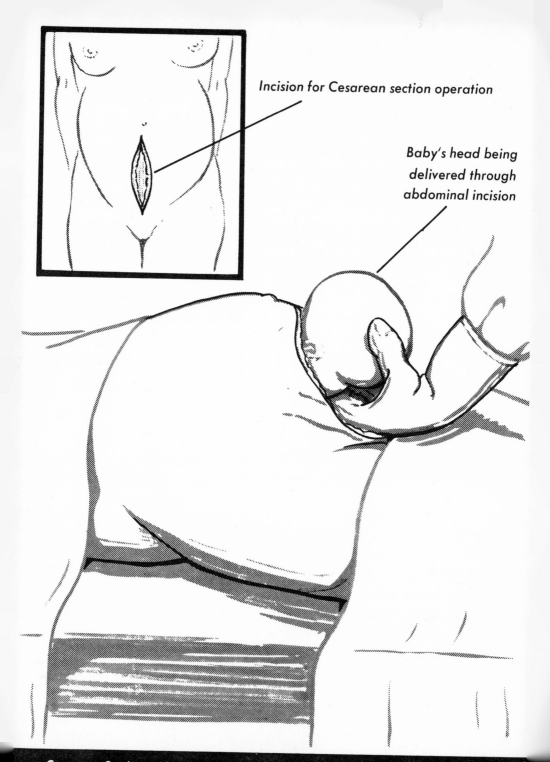

Incision for Cesarean section operation

Baby's head being delivered through abdominal incision

Cesarean Section. This diagram shows how a child is delivered through Cesarean section. An operative incision is made in the abdominal wall, the uterus is opened, and the child is withdrawn therefrom. The afterbirth is then removed from the uterus, the uterine wall is sutured, and the abdominal wall is closed in the same manner as after any abdominal operation. Cesarean section is a safe operative procedure.

A.D. The name has evolved from the tale that Julius Caesar was delivered by this method, but there is no historical substantiation for this legend.

If it is so safe, why aren't all babies delivered by Cesarean section?

In spite of the relative safety of this operation, vaginal delivery is still the safest method.

What are the indications for Cesarean section?

a. Disproportion, where the baby's head is too large or the mother's bony pelvis is too small to allow delivery from below.

b. Prolonged or ineffective labor which fails to respond to the usual methods of stimulation and where normal vaginal delivery seems improbable in a reasonable time.

c. Placenta praevia, when the afterbirth (placenta) lies in front of or below the baby's head. This is fraught with danger to mother and baby because of the danger of hemorrhage.

d. Abruptio placenta, when the placenta separates from the uterus before the delivery of the baby has taken place and where bleeding is too brisk to permit waiting for delivery from below.

e. Abnormal presentation, such as one in which the baby is coming down with an arm or a shoulder first and delivery from below is almost impossible without great danger.

f. Prolapsed cord, where the umbilical cord comes out through the vagina before delivery and delivery is not thought to be imminent.

g. Breech presentation in first pregnancies, where the obstetrician fears some disproportion betwen the baby's head and the pelvis.

h. Elderly women having their first baby, where some other abnormality exists.

i. Repeated previous stillbirths from unknown causes, where previous babies have died within the last few weeks of pregnancy or after the onset of labor.

j. Pre-eclampsia or eclampsia, where elevated blood pressure and other symptoms, with or without the onset of convulsions, make delivery urgent as a lifesaving measure.

k. Previous surgery, such as:
1. Previous Cesarean section.
2. Removal of fibroid tumors from the uterus.
3. Previous plastic operations upon the vagina, where delivery from below may lead to rupture of the cervix or vaginal structures.

l. Diabetes, where extremely large babies make delivery from below improbable.

m. A fibroid of the uterus or an ovarian cyst or other tumor which obstructs the pelvis and will prevent the normal passage of the baby through the birth canal.

Are all of the above indications for Cesarean section absolute?

No. It must be understood that there are many variable factors which will help the obstetrician to make his decision.

When will the obstetrician know whether a Cesarean section will be necessary?

This varies considerably. He may know on his first examination of the patient during the early days of pregnancy, or he may not know until after labor has been in progress for several hours.

Are there various types of Cesarean section?

Yes. There are many different technical procedures, but all types involve an abdominal incision, with the removal of the baby by an incision into the wall of the uterus.

What types of anesthesia are used for Cesarean section?

a. General anesthesia.
b. Spinal or epidural block.
c. Caudal.
d. Local novocaine anesthesia.

The type of anesthesia will be determined by the mother's condition and the preference of the obstetrician and the anesthetist.

Where is the incision made for Cesarean section?

In the lower abdomen, either a longitudinal incision in the midline or a transverse incision across the pubis.

How is the baby delivered in Cesarean section?

After the abdominal wall has been opened and the wall of the uterus has been incised, the surgeon's hand is inserted into the uterus and the baby is gently lifted out. The cord is tied off in the usual manner and the surgeon again inserts his hand and separates the afterbirth from the uterine wall. The incision in the uterus is then sutured with two layers of stitches and the abdomen is closed tightly.

How long does it take to perform a Cesarean section?

Anywhere from forty-five to sixty minutes.

How many Cesarean sections is it safe for a woman to have?

Usually, three or four. However, if the patient desires to have more children because of religious beliefs or other reasons, she may be allowed to have as many Cesarean sections as she wishes.

Can a patient who has once had a Cesarean section ever be delivered from below in subsequent pregnancies?

Yes. However, such a patient must be watched very closely from the very onset of labor, and the operating room must be alerted at all times to perform an emergency Cesarean section should a complication arise.

Is it true that most people who have had one Cesarean section will be delivered by the same method in future pregnancies?

As a general rule, this is true.

Is Cesarean section a painful operation?

Not particularly.

When does the patient get out of bed after Cesarean section?

The day following surgery.

Are special nurses necessary?

They are not essential but are helpful for the first few days.

How long after Cesarean section will vaginal bleeding continue?

For two to three weeks, followed by the usual discharge which ensues after a pregnancy.

Does Cesarean section interfere with subsequent menstruation?

No.

How long after Cesarean section will the first menstrual period appear?

In about six weeks.

Can a baby be breast-fed after Cesarean section?

Yes.

How long a hospital stay is necessary after Cesarean section?

About eight to ten days.

Does Cesarean section interfere with future pregnancies?

Not unless sterilization has been carried out at the time that the Cesarean section was performed.

How soon after Cesarean section can one safely become pregnant again?

About one year.

How soon after Cesarean section can one do the following:

Bathe	Four weeks.
Douche	Six weeks.
Drive an automobile	Five to six weeks.
Resume marital relations	Six to eight weeks.
Resume all normal activities	Eight to ten weeks.

POSTPARTUM HEMORRHAGE
(Hemorrhage Following Delivery)

What is meant by postpartum hemorrhage?

Loss of excessive blood following removal or delivery of the afterbirth (placenta).

What causes postpartum hemorrhage?

a. Failure of the uterus to contract following prolonged labor, overdistention of the uterus due to a large baby, or overdistention of the uterus due to excessive fluid within its cavity.

b. Retained placental tissue which allows bleeding to take place behind it.

c. A laceration of the vagina, cervix, or uterus which has occurred during labor.

Is postpartum hemorrhage dangerous?

The real danger exists in failure to recognize its presence or severity. A great deal of the danger has been overcome by modern methods of recognition and treatment and by the availability of blood for transfusion.

When is postpartum hemorrhage most likely to occur?

Either within the first few hours after delivery or, in delayed hemorrhage, several days after delivery.

What are the signs of postpartum hemorrhage?

Severe blood loss with signs of collapse and shock.

What is the treatment for postpartum hemorrhage?

a. If the patient is at home, she should be hospitalized immediately.

b. If she is in the hospital, blood is given immediately to replace the loss.

c. The cause must be established and appropriate corrective measures instituted promptly.

What specific measures are carried out to eradicate the cause of hemorrhage?

a. If it has taken place as a result of failure of the uterus to contract, medications are given to bring about contraction.

b. If a laceration of the vagina, cervix, or uterus is present, it must be sutured surgically.

c. If the hemorrhage has been caused by retained placental tissue, this must be removed manually.

THE POSTPARTUM PERIOD
(After Delivery)

When is the patient allowed out of bed after delivery?

Usually within the first twelve hours.

How soon after delivery can the patient eat and drink?

Fluids may be taken within the first four hours. Full diet is resumed within the first twelve hours. If a prolonged inhalation anesthesia has been given, fluid and food intake may be delayed.

What special garments are to be worn after delivery?

A good brassière and a firm girdle.

Is it common to require catheterization after delivery?

Yes. Difficulty in passing urine spontaneously after delivery is not at all uncommon.

How soon after delivery does the average patient have a bowel movement?

Usually, on the third day. A laxative is given on the second day. If there is no result by the third day, an enema is administered.

When do the breasts become engorged and tender if the mother does not breast feed her child?

By the third or fourth day.

If the mother does not breast feed the child, how are the breasts treated?

a. A good, firm support is worn.

b. An ice bag is applied if the breasts are painful.

c. Pain-relieving medicines and sedatives are given, if necessary.

d. Some obstetricians employ hormones to suppress breast secretion.

If the mother decides to breast feed her child, how soon will the milk start to come in?

By the second or, at the latest, third day.

How are the breasts treated when the baby is taken off breast feeding?

By giving medications such as epsom salts to induce dehydration, and by restricting fluid intake for a few days. If there is pain, analgesics and sedatives are given and an ice bag is applied to the breasts.

What is the treatment for tender nipples?

After the baby has fed, tincture of benzoin is applied in order to toughen the skin in the nipple region.

Should the mother continue to breast feed if the nipples bleed, crack, or become inflamed?

No. Under such circumstances, breast feeding should be discontinued.

How are breast infections treated?

a. By the giving of antibiotics.

b. By warm compresses to the breast.

c. If a localized abscess has formed, it must be incised and drained surgically.

Are the stitches in the vaginal region painful after delivery?

Yes. Some pain and tenderness is present for a few days. This pain is frequently alleviated by warm boric acid compresses and by the giving of mild sedatives.

1067

Do hemorrhoids ever develop after delivery?

Yes. They are a common complication and should be treated by the taking of lubricants to soften the stool and by the application of warm compresses or witch hazel to the area. Anesthetic ointments applied to the anal area may also help to relieve pain.

What is the average length of hospital stay after delivery?

This varies widely. Some obstetricians like to get their patients home as early as the third or fourth day; others hold their patients for five or six days.

How soon can one go out of doors after delivery?

Usually, about a week after leaving the hospital.

How soon after delivery can one return to all normal activity?

In approximately four weeks.

How long does vaginal staining continue after delivery?

The vaginal discharge is called the lochia; it usually continues for several weeks after delivery. It is not uncommon to have a vaginal discharge until the first menstrual period.

How soon after delivery does the first menstrual period occur?

Usually, within six weeks, but it may vary from five to eight weeks.

How soon after delivery may one shower?

Within two or three days after returning home.

How soon after delivery may one bathe?

Not until five or six weeks after delivery.

How soon after delivery may one douche?

After the first menstrual period has taken place.

How soon after delivery may marital relations be resumed?

After six weeks. It should be remembered that the first few attempts may be accompanied by pain or discomfort, but this will resolve itself within a short time. Adequate lubrication should always be provided.

How soon after delivery may one do housework?

This varies markedly, but most women begin to resume their normal household duties within two to three weeks after delivery.

Should the patient stay in bed after leaving the hospital?

No, but she should get into the habit of having a daily rest period for the first few weeks.

Is a special diet necessary after normal delivery?

No. A well-balanced diet is all that is necessary.

How soon do the female organs return to normal after delivery?

The uterus returns to normal by the sixth week. The breasts also return to normal size within approximately six weeks. The abdominal muscles seem to take longer to return to normal and may be lax and weak for several months after delivery. This condition can be helped greatly by exercise.

Is special treatment of the cervix necessary after delivery?

The cervix should be inspected after the first or second menstrual period following delivery. If it is then found to require treatment, it will be carried out by the obstetrician.

How soon after delivery is it safe to have another baby?

From a purely physical point of view, it is safe to become pregnant as soon as the effects of delivery have worn off, that is, within two months. However, the burden of caring for a newborn and the added household duties often make it advisable to space children more widely.

COMPLICATIONS OF PREGNANCY

What are the danger signs that indicate the possible onset of a complication of pregnancy?

    a. Increased swelling of the feet and ankles.

b. Sudden, marked increase in weight.

c. Disturbances in vision, such as disturbing "spots before the eyes" or double vision.

d. Severe persistent headache.

e. Pain in the upper abdomen.

f. Repeated vomiting.

g. Abdominal cramps, with or without bleeding from the vagina.

h. Vaginal bleeding at any time after the onset of pregnancy.

i. A marked decrease in the output of urine.

j. Repeated episodes of fainting.

k. Failure to feel the baby moving for more than one day, if this occurs after the sixth month of pregnancy.

Heart Disease in Pregnancy

Should a patient with heart trouble allow herself to become pregnant?

This will depend upon the type of heart disease, the presence or history of episodes of heart failure, and the ability of the patient to carry on normal activity without excessive fatigue.

Can most cardiac patients go through pregnancy?

Yes. Contrary to common belief, even damaged hearts are able to tolerate pregnancy.

What type of cardiac patient will have the most difficulty in carrying through a pregnancy ?

A patient who has had episodes of heart failure or one who has been unable to carry out ordinary physical activity during non-pregnant periods.

Is the heart patient managed differently during pregnancy?

Yes. Such a patient should be observed by both the obstetrician and the cardiologist. She is seen more frequently than the average pregnant woman and she is advised to rest more. If there are any signs of heart failure, the patient is hospitalized immediately.

Is delivery by Cesarean section always necessary for cardiac patients?

No. Cardiac disease in itself is not an indication for Cesarean section, although the cardiac patient does tolerate the procedure well when it is conducted properly.

Can surgery for rheumatic heart disease (mitral commissurotomy) help a pregnant woman?

Yes. In many cases where indications for heart surgery exist and the symptoms are on the increase, surgery becomes mandatory. This surgery can be performed as late as the sixth month of the pregnancy. Most women will tolerate the procedure of commissurotomy rather well and will be benefited considerably. (See Chapter 26, on the Heart.)

Can cardiac patients have more than one baby?

Yes, providing there is no evidence of heart failure and the patient is supported by the watchful care of both obstetrician and cardiologist.

Pyelitis in Pregnancy

What is pyelitis?

It is an infection of the kidney frequently seen during pregnancy.

What causes pyelitis during pregnancy?

Pyelitis is a bacterial infection arising from the bowel, the bladder, or some other source. During pregnancy, there is an abnormal amount of pressure on the ureters, which causes them to become partially obstructed and to interfere with free drainage of urine from the kidney. This situation predisposes toward the development of infection.

Is pyelitis serious during pregnancy?

Not usually. Treatment today, with chemotherapy and the antibiotic drugs, makes the disease easily controllable. However, if untreated, there is danger of permanent kidney damage.

Does pyelitis in the mother affect the child?

Not ordinarily.

At what stage of pregnancy is a woman most likely to develop pyelitis?

During the later months, when pressure upon the ureters is greatest.

What are the symptoms of pyelitis?

Urinary frequency, burning on urination, pain in the region of the kidneys or down along the course of the ureters. There may also be chills, fever, and nausea and vomiting.

What is the treatment for pyelitis?

a. Large increase in the intake of fluids.
b. The giving of sulfa preparations or antibiotics.

How long does pyelitis usually last?

Approximately three to four days.

Diabetes in Pregnancy

Does the finding of sugar in the urine during pregnancy always indicate diabetes?

Not necessarily. Lactose is often present in the urine of pregnant women during the later months of pregnancy, and this will give a positive test for sugar in the urine. Lactose in the urine does *not* represent diabetes.

How is diabetes diagnosed during pregnancy?

a. By the presence of glucose in the urine.
b. By tests showing an elevation of the sugar level in the blood.
c. By a blood test known as a glucose tolerance test.

Are all of these tests performed during every pregnancy?

No. Routine urine examinations are done for glucose. If a positive sugar test is found, then further investigation is carried out.

Are there certain types of women who should be scrutinized with particular care for the development of diabetes?

Yes; women who have had previous obstetrical difficulty, such as miscarriage, stillbirth, toxemia, or women who have had large babies weighing more than eight pounds at birth. Also, patients who give a family history of diabetes should be investigated with special thoroughness.

Is special treatment carried out for the potential diabetic?

Yes. She is more closely watched for signs of toxemia or other complications of pregnancy.

Are known diabetics a particular problem during pregnancy?

Yes. They must be followed by both the obstetrician and the medical specialist throughout the entire pregnancy. Control of the diabetic status is more difficult to maintain because of the presence and demands of the growing fetus.

In many medical centers throughout the country, it is customary to bring on delivery in a known diabetic about a month before full term. This is done to avoid the tendency toward toxemia and to cut down on the high loss of children which occurs during the last few weeks of pregnancy among diabetic women.

Must diabetics always be delivered by Cesarean section?

No. If they are delivered early, and all other things are normal, they may be permitted to deliver through the vagina. However, if there is any doubt as to their ability to deliver from below, these women are subjected to Cesarean section a month before full term.

What effect does pregnancy have on diabetes?

Pregnancy interferes with the ready control of diabetes, and therefore the diet and the insulin dosage must be altered frequently to meet changing situations. It is not uncommon for these patients to require periods of hospitalization at various stages of pregnancy in order to combat their diabetes.

What effect does diabetes have on pregnancy?

a. There is a high incidence of miscarriage.

b. Diabetic women tend to have excessively large babies with difficult delivery. Because of this, there is often a high percentage of disproportion between the size of the baby's head and the mother's pelvis.

c. There is a high incidence of toxemia of pregnancy, with increased dangers to both mother and child.

d. There is a high incidence of fetal death during the last months of pregnancy.

Toxemia of Pregnancy

What is toxemia?

It is a disease peculiar to pregnancy characterized by high blood pressure, damage to the blood vessels, the liver, and especially to kidney function. As a matter of fact, all body processes are disturbed in a woman suffering from toxemia of pregnancy.

What causes toxemia?

The cause is unknown.

How often does toxemia of pregnancy occur?

It is thought to occur in about 10 per cent of all pregnancies, but in the great majority of these instances the toxemia is mild.

What are the various types of toxemia?

a. Toxemia which is peculiar to pregnancy, such as pre-eclampsia and eclampsia.

b. Toxic states which are not peculiar to pregnancy, such as high blood pressure, kidney disease, and disease of the blood vessels.

What type of patient is most likely to develop pre-eclampsia or eclampsia?

Those who have had previous high blood pressure, kidney disease, or liver disease. However, many patients with no history of previous illness may develop toxemia during pregnancy.

Do patients with twins have a particularly high incidence of toxemia?

Yes.

Do diabetic women have a special tendency toward the development of toxemia?

Yes.

Pre-eclampsia

During what stage of pregnancy does pre-eclampsia occur?

Usually in the last three months.

How often does pre-eclampsia occur?

It accounts for about one out of three of all toxemias of pregnancy.

What are the symptoms of pre-eclampsia?

There may be no symptoms at all in mild cases, but in the more severe form the following symptoms may be present:

a. Nausea and vomiting.

b. Headaches.

c. Abdominal pain.

d. Diminished output of urine.

e. Disturbing spots before the eyes or double vision.

What are the signs of pre-eclampsia?

a. Swelling or edema of the face, hands, and most commonly of the ankles and legs.

b. Albumin in the urine.

c. Elevated blood pressure.

d. Unusual and marked gain in weight.

Is there any way to prevent pre-eclampsia?

The greatest part of prenatal care today is directed toward prevention of toxemia and early detection of the disease when it does appear. Routine examination of blood pressure, urine, weight, swellings, etc., are all done to detect early signs of toxemia. With early detection, preventive measures may be carried out.

What is the treatment for pre-eclampsia?

The following measures are advocated:

a. Salt and sodium intake is limited markedly.

b. Diuretic drugs are given to increase the output of urine.

c. Mild sedatives are given.

d. Drugs are given to bring down the blood pressure.

e. Hospitalization is advised if the patient fails to respond to the above measures.

f. Termination of pregnancy is advocated if hospital treatment is ineffectual.

What methods are used to terminate pregnancy in pre-eclampsia?

a. If delivery is anticipated in a short time, induction and delivery from below is indicated.

b. If a relatively short labor is not anticipated, a Cesarean section is advised.

What are the harmful effects of pre-eclampsia?

During pregnancy, there is danger to the baby and the mother for the following reasons:

a. Premature separation of the placenta with resulting hemorrhage is quite common in pre-eclampsia.

b. The disease may progress to true eclampsia with dangerous convulsive seizures.

c. Permanent kidney damage may result unless treatment is carried out conscientiously.

d. Infant mortality is much higher than normal in pre-eclamptic women.

What are the chances of full recovery from pre-eclampsia?

Treatment, as outlined above, will keep most cases of pre-eclampsia under control until the baby is delivered. After delivery of the baby, almost all patients recover quickly, with a return to normal kidney function and normal blood pressure within a few days. A small number of patients may take several weeks to regain normalcy.

Does pre-eclampsia usually clear up by itself without treatment?

No!

Does pre-eclampsia tend to recur during subsequent pregnancies?

Yes. There is a tendency toward recurrence.

Are there ever any serious after-effects of pre-eclampsia?

Yes, when there has been underlying disease of the kidneys or blood vessels before the pregnancy. In such cases, the elevated blood pressure, the impaired kidney function, and the damage to the blood vessels are further aggravated by the pre-eclampsia.

Are any precautions necessary after the woman with pre-eclampsia has delivered?

If kidney function, liver function, blood pressure, etc., have returned to normal, then no after-care is necessary. It is important, however, that these patients be checked periodically by their physicians.

Can a woman who has had pre-eclampsia permit herself to become pregnant again?

Before advising another pregnancy, one must weigh carefully the severity of the disease, the response to treatment, the presence of underlying permanent disease, and the number of babies the woman has had thus far.

The mere history of one episode of pre-eclampsia is not a contra-indication to subsequent pregnancy.

Eclampsia

What is eclampsia?

Eclampsia represents the end result of a pre-eclamptic state. In rare instances, it comes on spontaneously without evidence of pre-eclampsia.

How often does eclampsia occur?

In one out of eight hundred cases.

What is the cause of eclampsia?

The cause is unknown.

When does eclampsia occur?

Usually in the last few months of pregnancy. The most common time is just before the onset of labor, but it may sometimes occur during labor or in the first twenty-four hours after delivery.

What are the signs of eclampsia?

   a. Coma.
   b. Convulsions.
   c. Decreased or absent urinary output.
   d. Extremely high blood pressure.
   e. Large quantities of albumin in the urine.
   f. Previous signs of pre-eclampsia, with increasing headache, dizzy spells, vomiting, disturbing spots before the eyes, etc.
   g. Marked changes in blood chemistry.

Is eclampsia serious?

Yes. There is much increased risk to mother and baby when eclampsia exists.

How is eclampsia treated?

   a. By immediate hospitalization.
   b. By giving sedatives to control the convulsions.
   c. By giving fluids intravenously.
   d. By stimulating urinary output.
   e. By the use of drugs to bring down the blood pressure.
   f. By emptying the uterus as soon as the convulsions have been controlled for a period of twelve to eighteen hours. If induction is possible, delivery from below is carried out. If this is not feasible, then Cesarean section is undertaken.

What are the chances of recovery from eclampsia?

If recognized early and treated properly, the chances for complete recovery are good. If unrecognized or untreated, the results may end in maternal and fetal fatality. This is an important reason why women should make frequent visits to the obstetrician *during* pregnancy.

Are there any permanent after-effects of eclampsia?

If the eclampsia was treated early and effectively, there may be no permanent after-effects at all, providing that there was no pre-existing condition such as kidney or blood vessel disease.

Placenta Praevia

What is placenta praevia?

It is the presence of the placenta in the lower part of the uterus, below or in front of the head or presenting part of the baby. In this condition, the placenta encroaches upon the opening of the cervix into the vagina.

What causes placenta praevia?

The exact cause is not known.

What types of placenta praevia exist?

a. Partial placenta praevia, in which only part of the internal opening of the cervix is covered by the placenta.
b. Complete placenta praevia, in which the entire opening of the cervical canal is covered by the placenta.

How often does placenta praevia occur?

Approximately one in eight hundred cases.

What is the anatomy of placenta praevia?

The afterbirth is implanted at the edge of the internal orifice of the cervix, instead of higher up on the wall of the uterus. As the lower part of the uterus thins out during delivery and prepares for labor, the internal opening enlarges. This causes a separation of the placenta from the wall of the cervix, with resultant bleeding.

Can placenta praevia be prevented?

No.

What are the signs of placenta praevia?

The most important sign, and actually the only sign, is painless bleeding during the later months of pregnancy. This may vary from just a trickle of blood to a gush of heavy bleeding. The bleeding may stop immediately or may continue until it endangers the life of the patient.

How is the diagnosis of placenta praevia made?

By vaginal examination, with special attention to the cervix. The cervix is felt by the obstetrician to note the presence or absence of placental tissue on its inner surface. X-rays are sometimes valuable in demonstrating the presence of the placenta below the baby's head.

What are the harmful effects of placenta praevia?

a. There is danger of severe hemorrhage.
b. Placenta praevia usually requires early termination of the pregnancy. This may result in premature infants, with all the disadvantages of prematurity.

Is hospitalization absolutely necessary in all cases of placenta praevia?

Yes.

What is the most frequent time for placenta praevia to occur?

During the last two or three months of pregnancy.

What is the treatment for placenta praevia?

The standard treatment is Cesarean section. Delivery from below is advisable only in the rare case of placenta praevia. Prompt administration of blood must always be instituted if there has been severe hemorrhage.

What are the chances of recovery from placenta praevia?

With conscientious treatment, in the hospital, almost all patients will recover.

Are there any after-effects of placenta praevia following delivery?

No, unless the mother is markedly anemic from blood loss.

Is it safe for a woman who has had a placenta praevia to have another pregnancy?

Yes.

Does placenta praevia tend to recur in subsequent pregnancies?

No.

Abruptio Placenta

What is abruptio placenta?

It is the premature separation of a normally placed placenta from the uterine wall.

When does abruptio placenta usually occur?

During labor, before the delivery of the baby.

What causes abruptio placenta?

The exact cause is not known, but there is a close relationship between abruptio placenta and the various types of toxemias of pregnancy. In some cases, an injury is thought to bring on this premature separation of the placenta. In other instances, the sudden release of the fluid with the breaking of the bag of waters will cause premature separation of the placenta.

How often does abruptio placenta occur?

About one in five hundred cases.

What types of abruptio placenta are there?

a. Partial separation of the placenta.
b. Complete separation of the placenta.

1081

What takes place after the placenta separates from the uterine wall?

There is bleeding between the uterine wall and the placenta, and this may spread and cause further separation of the placenta.

Is there any way to prevent abruptio placenta?

Only by good prenatal care and the early treatment of any toxemia that may exist.

What are the signs of abruptio placenta?

Some or most of the following signs may be in evidence:

a. Vaginal bleeding.
b. Pain or tenderness to touch over the uterus during the last days of pregnancy.
c. The finding of an abnormally rigid or hard uterus on abdominal examination.
d. Nausea and vomiting.
e. Excess activity of the unborn child.
f. Absent fetal heartbeat.
g. Signs of toxemia.
h. Fainting, with a weak pulse and other signs of shock.

Is there always external bleeding with abruptio placenta?

No. The bleeding may be concealed and may remain contained within the uterus.

How is the diagnosis of abruptio placenta made?

By careful investigation of the patient's history and by physical examination, noting all of the above signs.

What are the results of abruptio placenta?

a. An extremely high fetal mortality.
b. Occasionally hemorrhage is so marked that it may involve the wall of the uterus and cause it to rupture.
c. The blood-clotting mechanism of the mother may be disturbed, so that dangerous hemorrhage may result.
d. Kidney function may be badly disturbed by abruptio placenta.

What is the treatment for abruptio placenta?

Treatment is first directed toward combatting any shock which is present. Blood replacement in the form of transfusions must be given immediately, if indicated. Pregnancy must be terminated, either by induced labor or by the performance of a Cesarean section. If the clotting mechanism of the blood has been disturbed, this must be corrected by the giving of substances such as fibrinogen. If the wall of the uterus has been badly damaged by the hemorrhage, a hysterectomy may have to be performed following the Cesarean section.

What are the chances of the mother's recovery from abruptio placenta?

If the diagnosis can be made early and the proper treatment is carried out promptly, recovery takes place in the vast majority of cases.

Are there any after-effects of abruptio placenta if treatment has been carried out promptly and adequately?

No.

What are the chances for a live baby in abruptio placenta?

This will depend upon the degree of separation of the placenta, the amount of bleeding which has taken place, the state of maternal shock when the separation occurs, and the speed at which treatment has been carried out.

Is there a tendency for abruptio placenta to recur with subsequent pregnancies?

Not unless there is some underlying disease.

Index

This Index lists the entries for this particular volume only. For a complete Index listing all entries in the entire four volumes of this New Illustrated Medical Encyclopedia, *see back of Volume Four.*